Changed Woman…Unchained

Life after AIDS

Faith, Dating, Career & all in Between

Written By

DeVondia Roseborough

Copyright page

© 2014 by DeVondia R. Roseborough. All rights reserved.

No part of this book may be reproduced in any written, electronic, recording, or photocopying form without written permission of the author, DeVondia R. Roseborough, photographer Tonya Patterson, or the publisher, Rasberrirose Foundation Inc.

Books may be purchased in quantity and/or special sales by contacting the publisher, Rasberrirose Foundation Inc. 704-906-5544, or by email atRasberrirose@aol.com.

Published by: Rasberrirose Foundation Inc., Charlotte, NC
Interior Design by: Lashawn Walls of Iziggy Promotions
Cover Design by: Dynasty's Cover Me,
Editing by: Complete Steps Publishing
ISBN: 978-0-615-97240-4
First Edition
Printed in USA

Acknowledgements

First, God gets all the glory for this story written for the masses because He first loved me and second He trusted me to do as He commanded: Go, Say and Do. For that, I am thankful for the opportunity to share my testimony repeatedly to all who care to hear. You have been the best Father a girl could hope for, I appreciate you watching over me, developing me daily, and shifting my atmosphere to a dimension, I was not ready for, yet you were patient enough with me to get to this point of not giving up on the journey.

To my loving children and granddaughter I love you girls so much and I thank God for you young women being in my life. Continue to keep God first and go higher than you expected because your future is great. I love you past infinity.

To my Aunt Geneva Hood and Aunt Sonia Funderburk I love you two very much and I thank God for the strength He has placed in you. Losing a child, I cannot identify with but losing a loved one, I can. My prayers continue to flow daily for your strength. Stay encouraged and I love you both.

My faithful executive assistant LaFewanda Baxter Robbins you are a blessing from God and I appreciate everything you do to help move US to the next level. God is moving. Let us ride.

To my Friends, family and loved ones please know I appreciate you in whatever role you play in my life.

To my Complete Steps Coaching and book cover designer Dynasty's Cover Me, thank you for making me look good. To my readers enjoy the message behind my life and never allow your circumstance to determine your future.

I dedicate this book to all the ones who said I could not do what I am destined to do. This book is for the ones who rejected me if I would have remained in your arms I would not know the power I possess. The words throughout this book are for the ones who talked about me, smiled in my face and said they had my back. This book is for you.

**This book is in Loving Memory of
Matto Ayim Nyiam and Davion Najee Funderburk
My loving cousins**

May you forever rest in peace know I love you forever.
Until we meet again "Handsdown... & BoBo"

*"Amazing how powerful the Holy Spirit is and what happens after you surrender...
Releasing, exhaling...breathing. Again"*

DeVondia Roseborough

I have been through many difficulties in my life and it was time for me to refocus on what is important, instead of what I had experienced. Yes, people overcome by our testimonies and I have shared and will continue to share what God has done for me. However, I am a changed woman now and I wanted and needed to move in another direction with my next release. For a day or two, I was stuck and unsure of what to write when it came to my life after AIDS. I prayed and released my thoughts and finally after watching a few YouTube videos celebrating the 42nd birthday of my favorite singer, Mary J. Blige on January 11, 2013, I wrote this caption...I'm a Changed Woman...Released. Released from bondage and low self-esteem that held me in a standstill for many years clutched like a tight fist I was released from negativity, a force that enjoyed my company and hated to see me strive for anything more than the environment felt I was worthy of. This book is about the woman I am now, the new DeVondia.

A memoir no, just a simple glimpse inside my journey since *Put It On Paper*, my first release based on my life before HIV and after AIDS. Changed Woman...Unchained will take you through a few decisions and choices after AIDS that were not all bad. You have to remember all things become new when you renew the mind and cleanse the heart but there are circumstances that try the flesh. I will focus on flesh forward; a mighty way to escape temptation of the flesh is to move forward in the flesh even when it is at war. This book written more so for women however, a man careful eye learn a thing or two as well on the challenges people face to push pass the pull that makes you stay the same.

My Secrets

Since my 2003 HIV diagnosis, challenged by God with a directive to go, say and do. Many days I regretted saying anything to anybody about my promiscuous lifestyle and many of the things I had experienced. If I had not, I would not have had the opportunity to meet the countless people, travel the world and make a difference in the lives of others. I wondered many days and nights tears in my eyes about how any man in his right mind want to spend the rest of his life with me. I have told just about everything there is to know about me and what I did would make any man walk pass me and not even carry on a meaningful conversation. I always felt that is the reason why I never had a relationship that worked. I felt if I had kept my mouth closed, no one would know and there would be a better chance at love if I were not as vocal. I had a man tell me one day, ***"If you didn't talk about it I would be with you."***

I felt like it was a no win situation because I had already been on TV, radio and appeared in print media so there was no stopping me now. All I could think of was, if I stop would he still want me or was it too late? The opportunity was bliss and as time was ticking, so was my age. I still managed not to give up hope that there was a blessing at the end just for me. During the process of waiting while distracted, there was opportunity to miss what was for me and I sometimes wondered if that special someone would come back around again since I was too busy in the garden of evil. There is no way to satisfy fleshly desires and expect God to bless you with the desires of your heart. I beat myself up walking around with my head up at the same time putting on a façade that I was the happiest person in the world diagnosed with AIDS. Not! My life was a living hell at times. I went to the salon and got the chicest hairdo, wore the highest priced clothes out of Ashley Stewarts and Belk, kept a pair of showstoppers on my feet and my face was beat with the best department store makeup money could buy. I made sure I was the life of every party and everybody loved me, but not how I wanted them to, or should I say that special man. My heart was yearning and my tears stained many pillowcases. I was often wondering and asking God when true love would come my way. I had skills in fixing other people's relationship issues, but I had a big secret of my own. I was more depressed at the thought of being alone for the rest of my life. Even my kids felt it was not necessary to have a man and that I needed to be alone. They knew my mood swings and the secluded events I slithered into when my heart was broken it affected them also. For a long time I decided not bring anyone around just because of how they felt.

As my depression sunk in, I began to focus on other things, like goals I wanted to achieve. I had visions of becoming greater than expected and bless abundantly so that I could be a blessing. However, something else wrestled inside of me, that I kept secret.

Deep within I struggled with this and did not want anyone to know. I had a fear of failure and was scared to death of success. I was terrified at failing in front of people and looking bad. Everything I put my hands on comes with great feedback and I could not stand to bring my bright ideas to the limelight fear of causing overcast. I was not having it, so I did not execute my awesome plans of action. I knew years ago, I had issues of anxiety and I was adamant about not letting anyone seeing me sweat. Fear paralyzed my ideas and my self-esteem, which gave me a sense of hopelessness. I spent more time thinking, instead of doing and when I started talking about what I wanted to do, I saw others put my ideas into fruition. Whether or not God gave them the vision or me forfeiting ideas, this was a wakeup call for me. God will allow people to do what you are destined to do right in your face because of your lack of determination and will power to do what He has gifted you to pursue. I was a great procrastinator. I would come up with these great ideas and sit on them, doodle on paper and fill up spiral notebooks and journal things I wanted to do. I had a great fear of releasing my inner power that required me to implement, but mentally I was not prepared and I had no idea how to refocus my mindset to believe that it was even possible. All of the stuff that happened to me in my life lodged so deep that it needed an outlet, a way to escape. I wanted so dearly for this not an issue. I came up with a quote years ago, **"Dreamers sleep...Believers cast Dreams"** When I would say this to other people I began to allow this to penetrate my being so that I would stop fancying my opportunities and start creating a way to make them come alive. Here I was a powerful woman to many yet I felt extremely small as if I could not make a difference. I felt like a failure. I do not blame these circumstances; they were factors to the delay of my outcome: Rape, toxic things, bad company, negative thinking and just operating outside of the will of God was and still is the bottom line, point blank period. Know that through Christ ALL things are possible and when I started to come to my senses that I am what I eat and all that comes in will come out, I knew it was time for a change.

The Importance Of My Words

We heard the saying if you do not have anything nice to say about someone do not say nothing at all. Well I had a few choice words of my own specifically for myself. "You are stupid." "How could you make this dumb mistake?" "You are ugly, "You are fat." I would literally look in the mirror and say these things and more, to me, with tears streaming down my face as if someone else was bullying me I was my own terrorist and I made myself feel lower than anyone could ever make me feel. I flipped the script and changed how I perceived myself. The devil was okay with how I felt and said but my Daddy, my Father, my Lord and Savior had an issue with that. I am fearfully and wonderfully made and I am the apple of His eye, how dare I tear down what is good. I had no other choice but to change my mindset and process positive words to influence my stagnation to a state of emergency. I was in need of deliverance from myself. We hear people needing deliverance from people and yes, I went through that too. Always needing validation and acceptance until one day, I acquired it. Who they were was not my concern because I had me that needed more attention. Once lifted, I was able to start moving from the bedroom, finally throughout my own home. What you feel about you is important and the words you use are a reflection of how your day and life will turn out. I could not do this alone. God had to be the forefront of this and I went to His Son Jesus for permission for deliverance. I desired to have higher self-esteem and confidence that did not come off as arrogant but affirmed I am somebody. Prayer is essential to moving forward and without it there is no way I could have gotten this far. I have read many books by authors who went through traumatic experiences and suffered from lack of self-worth. This made me realize a couple of things: I was not alone and that I did not want to be this way. I picked up a book from my local Wal-Mart by Joyce Myers titled *"Battlefield of the Mind: Winning the Battle in YOUR Mind,"* there was no doubt that this was what I needed. This book allowed me to grow, page after page as she included scriptures to cross-reference. In addition, I had my moment I must admit it took me a while to even open the book. Again, paralyzed by fear and procrastination of knowing, that on the pages of that book I would find the truth, and indeed, it was there. When I opened the book, I knew that there was no need in reading if I was not going to apply it to my daily living. Fasting, praying and studying the word more allowed my mind to change because I wanted it. How could I minister to others about self-esteem if I did not have mine in check? The flow began to circulate pure air that finally allowed me to breathe…I love me some DeVondia. I know that I am beautiful, I know no matter my waist size I am still fearfully and wonderfully made and no matter what people say or think it's what I thought is what was important. It was easier than I thought, but would not have known unless I tried. Glad I did.

I Have It In Me

Regardless of what the doctors said, what my naysayers believed or what I thought of myself I have it in me to do, say and go. I figured that the energy I used to do things that was against the will of God would necessitate just as much enthusiasm, so why not. Anything that is for me, I am going after it. No longer bound by heavy burdens and limitations that shackled my mind, saying I was not worthy or good enough to be or have. I am determined to triumph. Even in failure, lays an opportunity to reach the level of finishing what I start successfully. I have it in me, because procrastination has no say over when I will get it done or sneaking in my mind persuading me to do it later. Oh the feeling that came over me when I accepted the fact that it was okay to make mistakes, and that it was necessary for them to come out so all the refusal's has had their chance to shine. I could move forward after learning from what not to do, the yes's would prove it was worth it all. It was the best emotion that ever ran through me besides the sight of my children and granddaughter being born. The carnal woman in me wanted to accept what people thought. Pleasing them was more important than knowing what was within would not have a chance if I did not believe in myself I had it in me to be more than I was. I have it in me to make a difference in the lives of others and so do you. You have the opportunity to share your testimony with those bound by the same situation you were delivered. They need to hear from you but also need to see that it is real. Talking is simply saying something however, without any action there is no room for anyone to see the demonstration of what God can do when you surrender. What beautiful word surrender, is. Surrendering means to me, stopping everything that was not good, yet it-felt good, is cognitive of the importance of being in line for what is greater. Matthew 6:33 says *"Seek ye first the Kingdom of God; and all these things shall be added unto you,"* I had to stop searching for things to make me happy and ponder on what makes me better and turn everything completely over to God and trust that by seeking Him all things will be added unto me. Blessed to know that I had patience, confidence, the ability to thrive and make a difference and even love under the stuff that had me chained but these things would not be if I did not surrender. Surrendering offered me peace beyond understanding that even though they slayed me, I still have it in me to not act contrary to the word of God. I have what it takes to build up the next person. I am not limited to just managing my own personal growth because I dedicate my life helping others. Serving in a genuine capacity and being a blessing is what encourages me, simply because I have it in me. What lies in you?

Backing Up To See

Emerging into my greatness is a daily process and to see what was before me, I first had to trust that God was and is going to do everything He said He would do and surrender to the task of believing that it would happen. I generally am a loner, you would rarely see me with a pack of females hanging in the club, bar or mall. I roll in silence and make it my business to enjoy DeVondia. For about four years I hibernated from people, not completely, I went out and enjoyed friends every now and then but I turned down many opportunities because I was still in the not sure stage of my life. I was incomplete on what I wanted to do and my purpose was before me, but I lacked the motivation. One thing people need to learn about strong people, especially the ones that are always supplying the advice and know the right words to say, there is rarely anyone we can depend on. We find ourselves answering the call from many and when we decide to pick up to reach out no one is home. However, God said in his word, *"I will never leave thee or forsake thee* "Hebrews 13:5 (KJV). I had no problem casting my cares upon the Lord because His word says in Psalm 55:22; *He will sustain me and will not let his righteous fall.* Backing up and observing my mindset, my way of thinking-down to how I processed information was amazing to me. I was a fly off the handle type of person, the first thing came to my mind I would voice it without regards to feelings or what one would think. During this back up without sitting process, it allowed me to be more observant of my actions. I associated with a select few and began watching Oprah Life Classes and her Next Chapter series. I wanted to learn from people unlike me who had different skin tones and the ability to capture me where I was, but still connected with me on a common ground. I gained sight of my vision with my eyes open for the very first time. I could see. Sitting in my living quarters with a pen, a journal and the DVR set so I could really get into how to be the best DeVondia. I fell back but was in motion forward. From 2010-2012 I had a dry spell, my wilderness filled with why I am doing this to I do not want to do this anymore. I did not want to continue talking about HIV. I got tired of saying the same thing repeatedly and sharing my story with people who seemed not gets it. Then unexpectedly, I would get a text or inbox message telling me how inspirational I am and to keep up the good work. Every time I wanted to give up one of you saved me from giving in just because you reached out and encouraged me. I did not have many speaking opportunities and my book sales were down. I did not worry about bills, clothes, shoes or how I was going to eat because God takes great care of me and mine and even when we were down to our last He made a way. My pride would not allow me to reach out to anyone for help, but I managed to make a meal out of what we had and you can best believe my girls did not go to bed hungry. I was dealing with Fibroid Tumors for years but late 2011 they really came down on me and I ended up having surgery in

January 2012. I had a partial hysterectomy and was comforted of the pain and the periods! Thank You Jesus...During my six-week recovery time I had the opportunity to get in melody once again with God. My faith grew stronger depending on Him for healing and being free of what had me bound at least six days out of the month for twelve years. I was sitting back one day with my feet up resting and reflecting when He spoke to me; *"Go back to school"* For what? I am thinking and all I kept seeing was Life Coach this Life Coach that. As I researched, what a Life Coach was I started laughing because I was already providing Life Coaching services minus the pay. I prayed about it and asked God to reveal if this was for me. I even invested in a Life Coach to see how one operates and to sort out my own life. I needed some structure. My days overlapped between having a high school senior getting ready for college, a granddaughter on the way, my part time job and no social life besides Facebook and church, I needed balance in my life. I am thankful for meeting my Life Coach, Pat Kelsaw. She showed me three pieces of paper about what my life consisted of by simply telling her what I did daily. I almost had an anxiety attack when I saw how stressful my life was. Being here and doing this made my head spin just sitting there looking at the stuff that had me bound. I opted to sit down on some things and God told me the summer of 2012, *"Do not do any speaking engagements besides the ones you committed to and do not sale any books."* I was baffled at this but I had to trust God. After I had my daughter's baby shower and got my other daughter off to college,

I relaxed and was ready to do me. I remembered Pat telling me I was a *"Natural Coach"*, but I needed more, the basics, more understanding of what Life Coaching was and what my specializations would be. I pondered on it and continued researching schools as I waited for the okay to move forward. Money was an issue; my thing was waiting until tax season and getting it done then. God had other plans. For the first time in a long time, I was eager about fulfilling something without procrastinating. I opened my Facebook one Saturday morning and a woman out of Dallas sent me a message inquiring whether I had gotten my Life Coaching certification. I had not and she forwarded me an opportunity for a fast track certification and master certification in Life Coaching. Had I not gone for it then I would still be waiting on some money that I still have not seen for a class that I doubt would have had this great of a price. I thank you women for being a part of the plan, the divine opportunity to nurture my passion and that is serving others. During my classes, I noticed I was coaching myself out of the minor procrastination that still tried to rear its ugly head. I discovered my mindset was adjustable and I did not have to self-sabotage my opportunities and limit myself of better possibilities because of my fear of failure. Granted access and another chance to do something I found very helpful, I took a sabbatical. I did not go anywhere but to work. God allowed me to spend all my time with Him. No one knew where I was and what was going on. I was okay and God said it was okay. I even stopped answering the phone certain times of the day so I would not be disturbed. I needed to hear from God and the hustle and bustle of everyone in my ear having to be here and appointed this and assigned that and be was nerve wrecking. I needed a break from me, an opportunity to get it together before the New Year came in. October 2012 was my chance to sit back and do nothing but finish my certification and get permission to miss church. Yes, I said it. I got permission from God to miss church; I did not go for a month. I could not take hearing that I was doing too much. Do you remember the list I told you about with my Life Coach? I was overwhelmed with responsibilities and duties and still did not have time for myself, nor did I know what my next move was going to be. Prayer was the forefront of my sabbatical. I spent time alone in my room, which I was used to doing, and I pondered a lot. I heard answers to my questions and thoughts before they could come out my mouth. That is how amazing it was. I had a hard time asking people for things and I knew if I wanted to get ahead I needed some help. I needed an assistant to help balance all I had on my plate and a publicist to get my brand in order so I could make a better difference in the lives of women and girls. I stepped out on faith and God allowed me to come across a few publicists that sounded good. One almost got an agreement but God woke me up early one Tuesday morning and told me to do some research. I will say I was disappointed and even after speaking with them about my findings they were open about what was not true. I had to follow the sign of the Holy Spirit and rest assured I lucked up on a publicist for about five months. It did not work out but the time we spent working together was worth it and I thank God for her presence. I saw a post on Facebook one day from someone that said, "Be Your Own Publicist". I needed to work for me on my behalf and I am doing just that until the right one comes along. I put out a post on my social sites looking for an unpaid intern to assist me as an executive assistant. I received many responses but I ended up with the perfect one, LaFewanda Baxter Robbins. When I say God has given me the ability to stop, pray and listen and by being obedient I was able to hear His request unto me. I talked to my Pastor and First Lady about my absence and they truly understood. God even allowed me to purchase a new, dependable car. I was trying to decide if I was going to keep a 99, Lincoln Town Car He blessed me with a 2005 Chrysler Pacifica. Ain't God good? Of course He is! I pray that when it's time for my next mode of transportation, it's a Mercedes Benz and I'm crazy enough to believe I will drive what my heart desires and I am able to take care of what He provides me with. If had I not backed up to evaluate my present, analyzed 2012 and set my goals for 2013, I would not have received the blessing, I was counting on in 2013, wrapped in a bow in 2012.

Be still and see the salvation of the Lord. Wait patiently but move in the direction you see for yourself, because without sight of your vision you have nothing to look forward too.

What It Is Like Waiting?

I could scream at this chapter for this is something I deal with on a daily basis, so I must be honest with myself and continue to walk in obedience when it comes to the flesh. I had an addiction to sex. I liked it, I dreamt it, and I wanted it; but going about it the wrong way bought on disease and heartbreak. This in return caused the fear of being lonely and the onset of being more to a man than he was to me. Reaching out using careless whispers to intrigue the common man because the smarter the man the more game he had and we know the saying game recognize game. I knew I was not ready for a relationship with anyone, I just wanted company and of course, wanting to be held. Dealing with the emotions was one thing but having to put up with the demands of my body was another. I cannot speak for anyone else but I would feel the urge, the desire for sex but I had to renew my thoughts and focus on what was more important and that was pleasing God. 1 Corinthians 10:13 (KJV) ***"There hath no temptation taken you but such as is common to man: but God is faithful, who will not suffer you to be tempted above that ye are able; but will with the temptation also make a way to escape, that ye may be able to bear it."*** I listened to the words as I read them but I could not just read them without hearing what was being said, not only cognitively but my yearning flesh had to be saturated in the verses repeatedly. Repetitively, I recited the verse, but my body was saying otherwise. I even consulted women of God who had been in my quandary. They were as transparent as the words you are reading from me if not more. They broke down what they had to do. What worked for me was this; in the morning I woke up around three am, I was in my birthday suit and had gone to bed that night after drinking a glass of wine and having a good cry. I woke up, led to pray; lay before the Lord in repentance and forgiveness of my sins. Directed to the kitchen where my Olive Oil was. I had not blessed it yet so I did and began to pray. I remember someone telling me to anoint myself from head to toe and ask God to numb me down past the belly button. I blessed my house as I prayed. I touched the cabinets the appliances, the fixtures, the doorknobs, and I put on my robe, went outside, and blessed my property and everything on it from the mailbox to my car. I needed Him to know I was for real at surrendering and I know He wanted the same. After this long overdue worship service I felt relieved and satisfied but I knew deep down that the very thing that tempted me would rear its ugly head sooner than later. I met a guy who I fell for later, I do not think it was love, I just enjoyed the company he gave me. Well, long story shorter, I ended up breaking my almost year celibacy. I cried real tears, not because it did not work out, I went against what I had promised God. He had something special within him that noticed I was a woman of God but had things to work out. He never wanted me to compromise my walk and always told me to stay focused and on course for what God had for me. I did not want to lose him so I knew what to do to keep him coming back. Truth told that was not necessary. I was desperate for love and the affection and attention he gave me. Here I was starting all over again trying to perfect the walk of obedience. I knew if I went to church for every service in a day the more word in me what came out would be perfect. I stayed out of the club, refrained on too much wine, was mindful of what I watched on TV, and what kind of novels I read, and I figured I would be okay. I gave more time and dedication to reading and studying the word of God and watching Bishop T. D. Jakes and Joyce Myers on television. I watched No More Sheets by Juanita Bynum for the hundredth time and left with a different experience than the first. I trapped the temptation in many directions I knew how but the best way for anything unlike Him to flee is to say JESUS! I called His name many times to get my body to line up with His word. I shouted His name many nights for my imagination to get in tune with His scripture. I whimpered His name many days for me to conquer the fear of being alone because of my diagnosis with AIDS. I refused to settle. See back in the day, and I am sure nothing has changed, but overweight women known to have low self-esteem and they took care of their men. Not all of them, but there were a vast few who fell in the category along with underweight women and the fit and trim. In addition, I was no different. I made sure he looked like somebody when he stood beside me. I was critical on his shoe game, haircut and what he said in public. Not realizing that behind closed doors,

I was creating a monster. After many failed attempts to build a man for my satisfaction, I lacked the guidance of The Holy Spirit to lead me in the right direction. Preparing me first to be a virtuous woman and to recognize who was not for me when they appeared as wolves in sheep's clothing. I could not see the forest for the trees. I did not realize my branches bore fruit and I needed to nurture the ground I walked on with love, respect, patience, confidence and a different strategy, PRAYER! I never leave home without it and if I do, no matter where I am I reverence God. The waiting period is not like waiting for a bus or a phone to ring from that special someone. The waiting period in the beginning was frustrating. I did not want to wait; I wanted a man now. Someone to confess my love cooks for, draw baths, entertain, and wrap my arms around and all that I have to offer him and only him. I talked to myself knowing that I was a good woman but I forgot to confess to The Lord what I expected and needed in the man. I only wanted a physical body present without regards to what comes with relationships and how to work it out when the going got tough, because I was the one that would redirect my attention somewhere quick if things did not go my way. Forced, to be alone spending worthless evenings, nights and mornings with men that was not compatible with me. I had no clue how to date, never was I taught. I watched a lot of television and listened to friends as they spoke of what they experienced. I am sure I went on a few dates and was confident in showing respect for him and myself, however there were times when I wished I stayed at home alone.

I forced myself into solitude, a place of restoration, and a needed opportunity to know me on a different level, other than my need in having a man. I took myself out to the movies and restaurants, and treated myself to flowers. I ran my bath water sprinkled with milk and honey bubble bath. Being accepting of who I was and the calling on my life. I came to a breaking point saying aloud, If a man cannot accept the fact that I am vocal about being diagnosed with AIDS, running different businesses that will keep me busy and on the road, and that I love The Lord and He comes first, then family and my church, then he would have no place in my life! I had to convince myself this was true. I even tried myself to see if I was ready. How silly was that? I ended up in the arms of another man who had more baggage than I cared to lug. I was stronger in my faith but still weak in the knees. Of course, this did not last. I also had to recognize my ability to serve in the capacity I was destined. He also did not want to compromise my walk but the Bible speaks in Proverbs 7:21 specifically to what I was good at, **"With persuasive words she led him astray; she seduced him with her smooth talk."** I have one of the best talk games coming out of my mouth; however, I rather use it selling my products than seducing the life out of someone. I am persuasive, manipulative, arrogant, vindictive and downright thirsty with a mission that ends *with* **"I get what I want".** Sometimes it was more than I bargained for. Waiting means patience in knowing God will supply all your needs. He knows what we are in need of and in His word in Genesis 2:18 **"And the**

LORD God said, It is not good that the man should be alone; I will make him an help meet for him." Made just for me, and I am crazy enough to believe that my time will come when I am courted I am liked because of who I truly am, loved enough to warrant a bended knee, a ring and being asked will you marry me. The waiting phase is the time for preparation. Preparing to be a better woman was my first goal, but knowing who I was, was important to me so that I could learn how to be more humble. I needed to spend more time with God as I dedicated my time away from the ones in my life so that I could grow into the woman He requires me to be. What does it take to be the wife I longed to be first, stripping down the very fibers that made up the woman I was currently toting around in the very flesh that went with temptation rather than going in the opposite direction. I had to concentrate more on what the word said and meditate on it daily. I had to come to terms that I would have to submit to my husband and give up all control of being head of household. I would have to respect myself and him and lead a Godly life meaning, praying without ceasing and encouraging my husband by using the right words and not having rubber neck attitudes, and knowing how to solve issues without going to bed with wrath in our hearts towards one another. I had to be slow to anger and become soft spoken while adjusting my body language to align with purity, submissiveness, and be upright and righteous. There is so much to learn and I was willing to pull the plug on opportunities to hang out engaging in regular conversations and even dates to master the art of being a woman of God first as I prepare waiting for my king. I did and saw others state the word "Wait"... I found the definition wait and here is what stuck with me *"to remain inactive or in a state of repose, as until something expected happens (often followed by for, till, or until): to wait for the bus to arrive."* We cannot wait until a man arrives, we must be in an active state of prayer, fasting and preparation. First, praying to be the woman of God to the man of God that He is preparing for you.

Relationship With My Children...

If you knew me, you would know I love my kids to death and would do anything for them and I will not condone anything that is not righteous. I have been very hard on them because I felt like it was necessary. I refused to let the streets raise them or lose them to the dirty asphalt trampled on daily by misleading and tempting tactics to wear them down without an option is not a part of the plan. I think I did a great job as a mother protecting them from things and people, but I definitely did not do it alone. Prayer has always been the substance of all our family issues. I always had an open relationship with my youngest daughter Pumpkin; she is an opinionated woman, very inquisitive, highly intelligent and has a love for learning. She is my foot massager when she is home from college, my baby girl. My oldest daughter Pearl is a very smart and creative woman, vibrant personality and courageous. She has the ability to do anything she wants and has an unbreakable bond filled with love for her daughter, my first granddaughter, the apple of my eye with every muscle in her being. She is a spectacular mom doing all it takes singled handedly raising a daughter, with all she has. She and I bump heads a lot, she was my problem child, but now she is a woman that needs her own house for her and her child. After I learned she was pregnant, our relationship took a turn for the better. As a woman, my responsibility is to guide my daughters properly and I can admit that I was not always a perfect mother. I still am not the perfect mother however, I am better than before. I think it is important to lead by example when it comes to raising children. I could not continue doing things of the world and expect them to listen to me about things I did not want them to do if I was still doing them. I know how dangerous it is for our children to leave home seeing other people on the news not seeing their children return home is a knock at the door for any of us. Prayer is so important to me and being that my baby girl is away at a HBCU (Historically Black College or University) in North Carolina I must stay prayed up as I do for the one whose here in Charlotte. Being a role model for them is important to me. Even though I compete with other role models for my oldest daughter, I know that she loves me. Grabbing hold of them and never letting go no matter how old they get is vital to their success to being virtuous women. As I reflect on my past, I can remember the things I said and did when I was their age. Especially when they do an identical act, it makes parenting much easier. I know the right words to say and how not be emotional or erratic about certain things, but I will blank just like any other mother who knows they are doing something stupid. Some things I have simply thrown my hands up and said "Have your way Lord." I knew the drama I faced when it came to relationships and I use my transparency to let them know that mama has been there and done that and trouble does not last always. I see a bright future for my daughters and my grandbaby, Zion Nicole. My vision is to leave a legacy for them to be proud. They will want to lead the way when I am no longer able or when my body goes cold to continue with the vision. Setting them up for success begins with how I see success and anything positive that is accomplished is success to me. It is not about the money or the accolades it is about aiming towards a purpose and fulfilling the mission gracefully. I have a strong love for my daughters and I will get warm under my skin when it comes to them, but one thing for sure they love their mama. I thank God for the opportunity to share in their lives, to make changes and to hear the crazy stories they share with me. New Year's Eve 2013, Pumpkin asked me where I was going and my oldest daughter stood near and watched me as if they planned to ask me this. I told them as I always said every year since the first time they asked, "Church." They began to laugh and both of them said at the same time, "You always in church. Ever since you changed your life it's church this and church that." They started laughing but it hurt just a little for them to think this way. I went on to let them both know that I went through some things in my life and it was traumatic and usually those that experience a sickness, close death encounter or any life changing experience run for comfort. Thank God, it was God and not the arms of another man. From my response, I saw they understood, yet I learned that I needed some balance in my life. I was tipping my scales in many areas and neglecting others. I appreciated that conversation and I vowed to myself that I would do more fun things with them and for myself. Parenthood is a gift and blessed to right my wrongs from when I was not my best. I no longer had the urge to bring anyone around them that was unfit or worthy to grace their presence. I am responsible for building them up in what I do and whom I do it with is a reflection of them. I want them to see that I am a great woman and that God will use anybody. They recognized that I am a changed woman unchained from all that had me bound, because the love I have for them is solid.

Faith Of A Mustard Seed

I remember when I was in the hospital in 2004, Pastor Wendell Neal and his wife First Lady Ruby Neal an old classmate of mine came over to my hospital bedside to pray with me and I became saved on that day. I hate I cannot remember the actual date but I know it was in 2004, between January 2 and the 23rd that I gave my life to Christ. I remember him asking me if I had faith. I did and if I believed, I do. *"All you need is faith of a mustard seed."* He said. The size of a pen head, a small portion just enough to pull from. I activate my faith on the word of God but also use this scenario. I know Jesus performed miracles and I was one of them. Having a T-cell count of nineteen, 107-degree fever, pneumonia, seven blood transfusions, losing seventy pounds and... the doctors telling my mother there was nothing else they could do for me. Take me home and let me die. God had other plans for my life and because I activated my faith and trusted, He would heal and deliver me from my own lion's den. I have something I can look back on when things try to come down on me. I go back to my miracle and say with confidence, if God brought me through that He definitely can get me through whatever was trying to bind me up and spit me out. **Now Faith, is the substance of things hoped for, the evidence of things unseen, Hebrews 11:1 (KJV).** I moved beyond wanting tangible things I yearned for and prayed for total healing in my mind, in my body and for my soul. I had something down on the inside of me that loved serving others. I used every opportunity I could to help others by being obedient to all He put before me. Whether The Holy Spirit moved me to bless a man that was peddling for money or give a ride to a senior citizen who lives down the street from me to his daily recreation center outings. I have to trust God when He speaks to me. My faith activated through the word, but I know that with works is how I will see the fruits of my labor. We know that putting it into action is the definite way of seeing how God moves and growing more as He continues to prove He is God and God alone. Even when he does not I am crazy enough to believe what He keeps from me is okay because when inactivated faith falls on seedless grounds fruit cannot grow without proper planting, nurturing, watering or light. One of my favorite scriptures Proverbs 3:5-6 (KJV) ***"Trust in the LORD with all your heart and lean not on your own understanding; in all your ways submit to him, and he will make your paths straight.*** If this is not faith, I do not know what is. Trusting whom I cannot see, or touch, yet the feeling the Holy Spirit penetrate within lets me know He is real. I used to try figuring out His ways and how fascinating it would be to know more than what the Bible has to offer on God, but I know through prayer, and asking for the wisdom, knowledge and understanding that He will reveal all that is necessary for me to know. Gradually, I submitted to His ways and I am still grasping this concept daily. Nevertheless, I am flesh first and temptation ultimately tries to revisit. I am aware of a strong persuasion called conviction that will steer me back in line and straighten my path every time I appear to sway.

Toxic People, Places, & Things

    I refuse to have my character dismantled because of the company I kept, the places I went or the things I indulged in. I honestly almost lost many grand opportunities for being with the wrong person. It's crazy how I am writing this right now to music and one of the men that I was involved with, popped up in my mind because of a song that we enjoyed listening to, Alicia Keys' Unthinkable. I am so past him but it is amazing how things turned out, as I am figuring what my next chapter is going to be I was tempted by his good looks, his top-notch style, his amazing scent and top of the line conversations. It is what got me in the first place. I was engaged to a temporary opportunity. As a woman, I knew what I liked and the things that felt good usually were no good for me in the first place. Growing into who I am now I noticed that every twenty-four hours I am a stronger person, a wiser woman and I am better at being closer to who I am destined to be, simply by staying in my lane. I do not need to cross the freeway to have the same fun everyone else is having. I noticed that the ones who used to sit freely in my home when I smoked do not call anymore, invite me to as many cookouts or to house parties. Do not feel bad if you are reading this and thinking, "Oh, she is talking about me." I asked God to remove people, places, and things from my life that are not a part of the seasons before me and He has done just that. I love my sisters and brothers from back in the day and when I see them, I speak and show love but I understand that not everyone will meet me at my appointed destination. I did a detoxification that is still in effect. I still enjoy live music and dancing; I love watching a good movie with great people not worrying about motives or if I am going to be robbed. Picture that. I decided to take different risk instead of risky behaviors that will land me hurtful situations, unhealthy or in hell. There are challenges in life but the choices we make are usually the reasons for the issues we face. I knew that my time was now. The year 2013 was the year for me to see, feel and bless and there was no way I could make a difference being the same as the crowd. I separated myself. **II Corinthians 6:17 (KJV)** says, ***Wherefore come out from among them, and be ye separate, saith the Lord, and touch not the unclean thing; and I will receive you***. It hurt like crazy to see people who I thought cared for me not purchase my books, not support my events or even come to hear me speak. The saying you know who your friends are is very true, especially when The Lord starts blessing you; you see who was true indeed. I did not waddle there I just moved in the direction that was destined for my feet to journey and not detour. I no longer desired to be in the company of the ones who were not moving, still sitting around drinking, smoking and carrying on crazy conversations. I am not about that life anymore not knocking anyone on how they get it I am just not satisfied with living any kind of way. What example will I be if I minister to the youth and not live what I say? That is a hypocrite. I am human all day; I still get mad, but not as mad as before. Anything or anyone who is not flowing in a positive manner, I do not mind the separation. Being jealous of one's success is toxic and it is definitely a sin. The Bible states very clear that when someone rejoices; rejoice with them and the same when they mourn. It is highly important to not to be so caught up in self-gratification that we forget that it is not about us. I have seen many places and done many things, and I can mingle from the block to the boardroom and this life is far more pleasing than worrying about what I did the night before.

Flesh Forward

As I flesh forward, I know the only way I can fight this thing called temptation is to pray. As I pray, I am specific in my asking. I know I will be tempted many more times in my life than I care to be and I understand that. However, I ask God to strengthen me. I do not mind The Lord having full control over my mind, body and soul. I know that when I call on Jesus name anything that is not of Him has to flee. I have even been so bold as to want temptation to see if I would pass the test. God always provides for me and the feeling I get every time I achieve this allows my faith to grow stronger and tougher in The Lord. Prayer is my way of escape from what wants to bind me up and cause me to backtrack. I changed my hair a lot before going natural a couple of years ago and I decided to go even shorter. I wanted something different; I wanted to be free. I found when I went natural I was more attractive. Not by the looks and compliments, I received, by my beauty was no longer hidden behind a façade of pain and captivity. No, I did not get the big head. I am aware of how change brings on new opportunities for temptation to strike. I covered up my gray and covered the light blemishes on my face with MAC makeup and I am still the same DeVondia. However, temptation appeared the same. I gained a few pounds and working to get it off but temptation does not stop when I get on the scale. Each pound of temptation comes back just like it did the last time. Your phase in life may be stronger than the last or even open for discussion, but you do not want to flee. The very thing that tempts you most, will come back to break you or strengthen you. Just make sure you are a willing vessel to move the mountain that can very well crush you. I had this strong attraction to bad boys, it did not matter if he had dreads, was walking, living with his mama, or had no job with a strong hustle I knew what I was in need of. Now, I have a newfound love for a grown man, in a tailor-made suit, a professional and God-fearing man, who is well rounded, and culturally diverse, with a love for family, someone striving towards a level of expectancy in his life. I do not mind jeans or even Jordan's on his feet every now and then but he has to be fit for a queen. There is no need in dumbing down your conversations to appease an opportunity with looks, I desire a man of substance. I was talking to my barber Quarter one day and we both agreed that it was time to bring dating back into our lives. We messed up engaging in sex before getting to know those we have connected with, which has led to many regrets. Dating allows people to interact on a get to know basis instead of acting off emotions one may bring because he smells good or looks better and it may not be good at all now you have gone and fell into the devil's playground with less and gained more stress by not courting in the first place. I fell out of sync in the dating world because of this. I did everything out of order. I knew it was time for me to do better so that I could be in position. Trying to be a kept woman is more work than anything else is my opinion.

Recently, as I thought to myself I needed to get away from my normal routine so that a man could ask me out. People kill me, waiting on the Lord and single. You can be a kept woman. However, being in the fetal position hoping for a man is not the way. Get up, dress up and show up woman of God!

Where Are They Now?

When I went in the hospital in 2004 I was nearing death, let the doctor tell it, but God had another plan for my life. I remember my mom telling me that she did not know I had as many friends as I do. My friends are supportive and I believe they love me very much, but I must be honest, I do not see them much anymore. When I realized that things had changed, I began to cry.

I was on Facebook one day and saw a post where someone shared a picture of her friends enjoying themselves on a night on the town. I had my cousin to contact my friends that were there with me from the beginning so we could meet and discuss where we were in our lives, but also how I felt about us not being as close as we used to be. I will be honest, I dropped the ball and I was in my feelings. I never followed up and kept doing what I knew to do; thinking all was well as I kept them and their families in my prayers daily. I know people are busy with their lives, enjoying loved ones, working and some may feel because I attended church that I had changed. I have, but guess what; it does not take away from the fact that they are my friends. I love old sayings because they remind me of what I am not going through. This one fits right in. You know who your friends are when things get rough. Lord knows I am thankful for the love and support my friends showed me during this trying time in my life, yet what happens when things are going all right. I will admit that I am not doing my best at being a good friend either.

Caught up in my world of going, saying and doing that I fail to stay connected with my girls. We have passed the stage where we sit up in one another's houses on a weekly basis drinking, smoking, laughing and enjoying ourselves. We have matured to a level where we can meet on a monthly basis to have a glass of good wine, some laughs accompanied with a good meal. I need my friends to survive and I know good and well they feel the same about me. Friendship means a lot to me and the ones God blessed me with are amazing. They stick by me through thick and thin. They love me regardless of the choices I make and they are trustworthy. I feel at times that they hide things from me in fear of me becoming "Mama Dee". This brings a smile to my face as I sit here laughing and write this, many of you don't know that I was held back one year and my mother retained me a year because she felt I was not ready to go to the next level. My, my, my-that is a chapter heading.

I was always older than my friends were and for me it meant being wiser because I am the type of person who possess a trait that I admire. I am a critical thinker that actively listens and provides sound advice. They respect my words and many appreciate the encouragement I deposited in them as we were growing up. I cherish my friends and I would love for this to be a revelation for those who are reading this. Appreciate your circle, keep them close, and let them know often how much you care. If you have to set an alert on your phone to remind you, do it. If they cross your mind, call or text and tell them, know you were thinking about them. Do not ever let the day go by and you are thinking of a friend and you neglect to reach out because you were too busy. Form a habit in communicating with one another. Friendship makes the world go round just like family. Honor your friendships by getting on each other's calendars and make it your business to be accountable for your role as a friend. To my loving and caring friends...Angela Bush, Tiffany Barringer, Melissa Gibson, Wanda Hughes Glenn, Theresa Kimble, LaShawn Walls, Shawn Weddington-Spears, Toya Adams, and Kim Williams. We go back to the sounds of Ready for the World, the Whop hair do and doing the Roger Rabbit at Cochrane Middle School on the bridge, please if your name is not listed do not feel slighted or offended. These are my backbones right here, they have been with me since before my kids and Facebook. To Toya, I am glad the misunderstanding understood, the tears were dried and the forgiveness was accepted. Continue ladies never allow anything or anyone tear us apart. I love you ladies forever, no matter what.

He...Him...Them

Salvation was a major decision, staying saved is a daily chore. It is hard work to stay as close as I can to being Holy. Trouble is easy to get in but hard to get out. I slipped, fell, hit my head, got up and started the process over again, if I failed the test. When God gets to blessing here comes the messing, it never fails. You already know that my mess comes in the form of that temptations of the flesh; ole sexy tall black man with beautiful skin smelling like a bag of money...Dirty. Knowing good and well if I slip up I am doomed to get the wrath just as quick as the decision I made to commit the sin. I remember a time when I was dating this guy who I felt was right in so many ways. He was eyeing me from afar and he let me know this. One night I had a nice relaxing night out and he kept my glass full at an event with Moscato. I was feeling like a million bucks, light on my feet and the more I sipped the better he looked. We started to spend time with one another and our great conversations soon led to daily talks, laughter, lunch, dinner and a movie or two. My favorite time with him was watching the NBA playoffs. He is a Bulls fan and I am a LeBron fan. Let me clarify because I do not really have a team that I am a fan of LeBron. I admire him for being a young black man with a mind to do everything possible to make his mother proud.

I shared in *Put It On Paper*, about my abortion I had when I was in my late teens. When I became pregnant with my third child, I wanted her to be a boy so bad. I never had a son and I felt the baby I aborted at 12 weeks was the son I never had. Nick Cannon came out with a song titled "Can't I Live." When I heard the song for the first time, it broke me down to my knees asking God to forgive me and apologizing to a baby who could not hear me. I felt every word was to remind me I did not have to do it, but I did. It is something about LeBron, it is not attraction at all, it just makes me wonder what my son would be if he had a chance. I do not know if he was a boy or not, but I felt he was.

    I enjoyed the time I spent watching sports with him. Finally, someone to share my time with who was not afraid of what people thought or said. I was not aware that it was not okay for me to be in the company of him until I asked someone about him separated. "He is still married and once his divorce is final then it is okay." They said. I was done. The relationship dissolved and when we finally spoke months later and what feelings I had, were no longer there. I stayed to myself for about seven months after my surgery in 2012. I spent my days reflecting during my recovery. I finally visited one of my favorite eating spots, Sunset Soul on Beatties Ford Road in Charlotte, NC. Now if you are ever in the city, stop by Angie's Diner or Sunset Soul and support these black-owned businesses, I promise you will not regret it. As I was waiting on my food a dark skinned medium built handsome man, come in with his cousin. I noticed that he kept looking at me and smiling. Finally, he asked was any of the guys in the restaurant were my husband or boyfriend because he did not want to be disrespectful in telling me how beautiful I was. I smiled and shook my head no. We became instant friends and we quickly began our middle-school check in's and the daily conversations of getting the skinny on his life before me and mine before him. We decided to have our first date, but here I was nervous as ever. I said it before and I will say it again, I did not know how to date. Everything out of order I was a tad bit confused. There is no shame in my game because I am sure some of you feel the same way. Our date began with dinner at Hooter's in Downtown, Charlotte, NC. We enjoyed sipping on Sangria, eating chicken wings, while enjoying one another as the night air encouraged our exploration of one another. Following our dinner, we walked through the city while still engaging in casual conversations. When I say I had a good time, believe me, I did. Once our night ended he went home and I went to my dwellings with a smile on my face and thoughts on my mind to reassure me he was a guy I could get to know until I found out that the baggage he toted outweighed mine. I instantly had to fall back. Not only was he walking around with suitcases full of past relationships and insecurities, he had low self-esteem as well I did not have time for that! I longed for an opportunity to be in good company and here after so many dates, and conversations the real appears**. "Don't nobody have time for that!"** in my best Sweet Brown voice.

If I was no good for a man when my self-esteem was low, you know he was not any better for me. I threw my hands in the air and waved them as if I really cared about the direction in my social life. I knew that something was still on me that attracted the same outcomes. I met a nice man on Facebook a few years ago not long before he married and we had great conversations that lead me to know that there are still good men out here. He truly loves his wife and kids and I appreciate his honesty when it comes to how I should fit in when the man for me finally arrives.

TIPS TO SURVIVE IN A RELATIONSHIP:

- Never tear your mate down. Build them up and encourage them no matter what;

- Be honest with yourself if you are not ready. Do not force a screw to do what a hammer is equipped to do;

- Be you. Do not allow the representative to be more attractive than YOU;

- State your cause. Ask yourself, are you dating for fun or for marriage? Do not scare them off however; do not hang on because every GPS has a destination;

- Balance everything you have going on effectively. You cannot afford to lose focus if your emotions are off guard;

- If God is not in the midst do not entertain the season with reasons why later.

Behind Closed Doors

I often wondered when it is going to be my turn. During April 2013, I saw quite a few of my friends post on Facebook "I said yes" or "She said yes". The holidays come and I am alone, just like now. Today is Mother's Day and I am sitting in my room with the door closed and tears running down my face. I received two special shout outs and they were from someone else's husband. Good friends of mine who saw fit to show me some love today. I am so happy for them because they are extremely happy within their relationships and they tell me all the time to wait patiently, when your time comes just be ready. Behind closed doors, I talk to myself. I ask DeVondia questions and she answers back. I listen to a lot of music and I enjoy all genres. I stare at the walls with my head back while my arms rest on my forehead and at times warm tears trickle down my cheeks. One day while I was alone, I decided to light a candle and turn on some music. I began writing my thoughts on paper and before I knew it, I had ideas for three books and branding improvement for my company. I contemplated on a lot of wording. I was trying to figure out what I wanted to say without offending anyone or compromising my walk with God. Behind the lock and key, I went back and forth mentally on continuing with the outspoken HIV stuff. Sharing my story, educating others in the community and being positive with a smile was burning me out. I recently told someone that I do not like doing this; I do it because God gave me a directive.

However, I love doing it because I care about people, if that makes any sense. Behind closed doors, I will say a few choice curse words. Yes, I am like Peter, but I pray daily for forgiveness with help with seasoning my speech. Behind closed doors, I am very imaginative; I create opportunities. As I look in my phone contacts, I realize the people who are imperfect to my reality deleted. I look at myself and examine my exterior as I try to figure out what is wrong with me? Why can I have what everyone appears to have? Then one day I realized that people only wants you to see what they want you to think is all-good for them. It can very well be peaches and cream but for sure, I know there is a season for us all. Behind closed doors, I can allow my breast to rest without a bra and snack in my bed as I dry tears listening to a song that reminds me of a love that I once knew. Now when I open the door is a song that best describes me by Deon Kipping, "I Don't Look like What I've Been Through." Google that song and while you are at it search me to.

Rejection

The worst feeling in the world, told NO! Honestly, no one rejected me where it hurt my feelings bad, since the first time that I spoke on it in *Put It On Paper*. You want to know about it, I suggest you get the book. The people I had an attraction to let me down in a gentle way. In a way, that made me accept knowing it would not work. Now, I am the one who does the rejecting. I find myself limiting my opportunities because of how others have treated me. Therefore, I keep my guard up as if three pit bulls surround an electric fence with a sawed-off shotgun loaded to protect the feelings of the one and only me! With the diagnosis, it comes with pros and cons and when it comes to rejection, I sabotage myself due to my behaviors, which leads the individual to pull away. Dangerous as it may be, as a woman who is aware of her worth, I am destined to believe that God has a soul mate just for me. The thought of a man hurting my feelings is far worse than the experience itself. Trust me, I have been through enough heartache and heartbreaks to know what it feels like to hurt by the one you love, however the fear of premature misperception is not what you want to experience. What is premature misperception? Glad you asked. Premature misperception is an assumption in thinking on someone else's behalf without regards to their honest thoughts and feelings for you. You take on your emotions and intertwine them with your perception and there you have it, a premature misperception. Never allow your mind to think the thoughts of others. Training your mind to think in this way can prevent you from opportunities from the very one who may feel the same way you do and here you have self-sabotaged yourself all over again. Rejection came along accompanied by a combination of things I experienced in my past. For one, my dad not being the father I felt he should have been in my life left me feeling abandoned and rejected at the same time. Raised by a beautiful single woman who worked for hers, I never saw my mother in a toxic relationship. For me to have been involved I wished I would have taken what she displayed morally and developed it into my character years ago. Rejected in relationships was not my only problem. I feared being told the word no. Whether a job, a book deal, collaborating with others to make a difference, or someone disagreeing with an opportunity. I feared the word no sounding off between my ears and then having to go to the next person and wondering if they would say the same. Driven to do many things alone to neglect the sound no coming from anyone I purposely orchestrated, community events, book signings, even going out. I got tired of hearing people say they did not have anything to wear. Rejection made me feel a feeling of lowliness creating a close to sick sensation in the pit of my stomach that had me regretting at times being born. I am so glad I changed my perception of thinking. As I sit here and type this, I remember wanted by men that were already in relationships. I know it sounds crazy but it is my truth and I am sticking to it. I tell people all the time, do not let the AIDS diagnoses fool you thinking that he will not because he will, if I let him. That is the key if I let him in.

As women we need to know that if we are being pursued in a way that will take us out of character and degrade us based on the fact that he is involved or married, we lose more time on being courted ourselves by the very one who is sitting back watching our every move. In addition, trust you do not want to be before an angry God! I have asked several guys why even got married knowing you are going to cheat, Not necessarily with me, but these are conversations that I have engaged in with some of my homeboys who trust me with a lot of information on how they are feeling and what they are experiencing within their relationships. You know for some, they think I have a safe face, no one would think we were messing around. You get the picture. Stay connected to what you know is right, do not lose focus and stay ready at all times because even the best of the best are told no. Everything and everybody is not going to agree with you or want to be what you would have them to be so it is vital that your mind lines up with the word of God and your heart follows. I love this song, "What God has for me it is for me" Yet I wonder when mine will come.

My Highlights

Let me tell you about some grand opportunities presented to me since 2008. I released *Put It On Paper* January 23, 2008 and it has been MY best seller ever since, not New York Times, but mine. I love the book I truly do, but I have to admit, My Last First Kiss was my best written and it is far more creative, at least in my opinion. Nominated in 2009 for the Steve Harvey Hoodie Awards for the Best Community Leader category but I did not make it as one of the top four finalists. The Hoodie Awards then, now called The Neighborhood Awards. It is an opportunity for the community to nominate the best of the best in several categories, ranging from The Best Soul Food to The Best Nail Salon. In 2010, nominee and finalist awarded me an all-expenses paid roundtrip to Las Vegas, which included room accommodations at the Mandalay Bay Hotel, passes to all of the events and the opportunity to meet the celebrity presenters. I have never been star struck, but when it comes to meeting Mary J. Blige, I promise I will pass out. I met some great people from the airport to the stroll I took at six in the morning down Las Vegas Boulevard. I hold that memory dear to my heart. So many people thought of me to represent my city and state running against other individuals from St. Louis, New York and the finalist from New York won, but I still was a winner. Sitting in the third row from the stage and the big camera had my face on the big screen numerous times smiling and looking like a million bucks. I had a ball snapping my fingers to the O'Jays, Angie Stone, and my girl Fantasia. She came out to perform after her alleged suicide attempt and was on fire. During her song, "Bittersweet" I stood up and sang the entire song. I love music and I have to be on my feet when something sounds good to me. Everyone else was sitting down and she acknowledged me before the crowd by saying, *"North Carolina I see you."* I love that girl and I wish her the best and I thank God for the opportunity to share this moment. In 2011, I received a call from a producer from CNN wanting to do a story on me. Because I could not get anyone to commit to a time to have, groups of kids listening to me speak or a group of women they opted to feature me on HLN with Robin Meade's Breakthrough Women segment honoring women doing great in the community in which she lives. This was a grand opportunity nationally seen for what I love to do and that is serving people. In 2012, told that my oldest daughter was pregnant. I was not surprised, believe me, a mother knows. When it finally came out, I was ecstatic about becoming a grandma for the very first time. Whom will she look like and what would her name be, were some of the conversations my daughter and I shared. I am grateful for my friends and family who supported her and have been there since the beginning. Zion Nicole was born at 12:33 pm July 31, 2012 weighing 6 pounds and 10 ounces, the splitting image of her mother at birth. I love that little girl with all my heart and I sing to her these words. *"I love you so much I love you so much I love you more than I love my own kids."* Ha! It is true, wait to you become a grandparent. I love my grand baby more than I love my own kids, a figure of speech. It is a different kind of love. Especially when she looks into my eyes, staring at me forming a beautiful smile as she rubs my face. During the same year, my youngest daughter graduated high school and two months later, I had the esteem pleasure of escorting her to North Carolina Central University for her first year majoring in Criminal Law. The ride began early one Saturday morning with us holding hands praying for a safe ride, a positive year with protection and the blood of Jesus pleaded over every situation and circumstance in advance. When we arrived, she picked up her keys and we had help unloading and taking her things up to her residence. I took a little nap before I hit the road to travel two and a half hours back to Charlotte. Not far, but far enough when you cannot get to her when she really needs me and I thank God she never had to make that call. I thank God for not having to hear her crying on the receiving end for anything. As I got up to leave she started crying. I looked at her and said what is wrong? She wanted to go back home she said. I talked to her about how hard she worked to get here and if this was what she really wanted to do. *"Of course, not"*, she said, so I knew I needed to hang around a little while longer. I decided to take her out to eat and let her see where the nearest CVS and Wal-Mart were. We were walking around Wal-Mart and people were calling her name from everywhere. My daughter was a flag girl captain for her high school, at West Charlotte High School and participated in competition in Durham and other cities up and down the East Coast. I reassured her that she was going to be just fine. When her friends called to let her know they were on their way to move in their residence halls, she had no problem letting me go. I put on my big girl panties, my panties are big anyway, but I did not let her see me cry. I cried down the road all while praising God for the opportunity to be in the number to witness this awesome milestone in my daughter's life. Never listen to words that say you can't, you shouldn't and you will never; it is highly important to believe that what God has for you is for you and the events that you will share are for you and you alone to savor and thank Him for. Even the simple things deserve recognition. Celebrate yourself and others around you.

Self-Care

My health had been great thus far, but during the early part of 2011, the virus showed its ugly face in my test results. My medications were not working according to plan and I became resistant to them. I switched to a different regimen that has been working well for me and back to undetectable level of the virus claiming by His stripes, I am healed, regardless. After my partial hysterectomy I started to relax a little more I guess because I had no other choice. I paid more attention to the food I was putting in my body and was definitely looking forward to the retreat with my coworkers in Durham, NC at Avila Retreat Center. The retreat center runs by nuns and the cottages on the property, not what I expected. I had twin beds to choose from, no TV or a radio, What the What. I had to change my mind very quickly on being okay with a graveyard for families who could not afford to bury their baby's right behind me. A beautiful, yet somber sight, adorned with teddy bears and balloons embellishing the graves of tiny souls who did not have a chance. I love the fact that the grounds are sacred displaying the Crucifixion of Jesus on the cross and a beautiful lit statue of Mary holding Jesus after taken down from the cross. This was always a nice get away to clear my mind, to release stress and more importantly to hear the voice of God. Self-care is very important for everyone however, when you are living with any life changing disease it is imperative that individuals take better care of themselves. I found myself at a point of always running, doing and helping others when I needed time to myself, my house occupied with no welcome to hold. Self-care to me is being in the right frame of mind and not allowing anyone or anything distract me from my purpose, eating clean and healthy foods, drinking water, exercising and no stress. Of course, I have to take my medicines twice a day and trust that God will do just what He said He would do. I desire total healing whether on this side or the other side. Until then, I will continue to claim by healing and doing what He says is a sure way to receive the desires of my heart. I made up my mind and decided I was going to lose the weight I gained. I was nearly 260 pounds; however, between being five foot nine, and a girdle, I carried it well, but it was not healthy. I received some news that I was pre-diabetic and I immediately went into weight loss frenzy. When I went back to the doctor, I had only lost a few pounds and my doctor insisted that I would be going to the diabetic clinic for classes on how to take care of myself, but God said no. My test came back great and He allowed me hear her tell the nurse that I did not have to go. God is so good. I did not want to take any more chances so I joined the YMCA close to my house and worked out faithfully five days a week for an hour and a half. I lost twenty pounds during that time and striving for about seventy more. I joke a lot; hey, I was the class clown of my senior class. One of my church members told me one day, *"Sister Roseborough, you been dressing up a lot here lately, you have a boyfriend?"* I told her when I testified in church at an afternoon service I had no boyfriend, I could finally wear my clothes and I want to be right. Having a pretty face and a Michelin Tire body is not going to attract many opportunities for a date; it is only my little joke, do not bend out of shape. Big girl's rock but they sway even better with a toned body. Self-care helps me to love myself more than I did before, without limitations. The things I can fix I have the willpower to change my mindset so that it aligns with my agenda as I proactively and strategically put it on paper and hold myself accountable for every nook and cranny. Taking care of myself leaves me in a better position to tend to the needs of others because we have heard time and time again, *"If I am no good for myself I'm no good for anyone else."*

Facebook

    I recall opening up a message on Facebook one day and my friend Titus Broom told me how much he appreciated my daily post and titled me the "Facebook Oprah." I enjoy inspiring individuals and many of you that are reading this need to know just how much you supporting me encourage me as well. Your support has encouraged me in ways that you will never know. There were days when I wanted to give up and not continue, but your inspiration is one of the things that helped me. I wanted to literally give it all up and move forward in doing me, then a message would appear at the right time to bring me back to reality, because my doing me would definitely not be pleasing to God. There are so many hurting young girls and women whose lives I influence daily. I wanted to make sure that my guidance in leading them would be a fossil forever embedded in their hearts. What disturbs me most about Facebook is when women degrade themselves for attention; you know, taking half-naked or fully naked pictures and post them on our social media pages for everyone to see; searching for the satisfaction of a like or a comment but get upset when someone demeans their character for the selfless act that they just committed. I cannot understand for the life of me why people argue over someone not accepting their friend requests. There will be that one that do not have a Facebook page but can tell you everything going on with someone else's. Fighting over what is about them being a busy body. Facebook beef is what I call it and cannot bust an orange down with a potato peeler, ridiculous and starving at the same time for attention. As women, we have a moral standard to set an example in the presence of people, in the privacy of our homes and on social sites. I hate that our youth already have to deal with the perception of role models seen on TV, their own parents, aunts, cousins; friends are acting out of control. It is a saying I hear all the time, "Meet them where they are," well what if you do not feel like it. You have a choice to either put up with foolishness or not. Personally, I would rather be educationally entertained any day than disappointed. In short, Facebook has given me a lot to be thankful for and it comes in the support of you. Thank you for all of your love and encouragement, I love you all.....DeVondia

Fear

When it comes to relationships, they are important to me. I will admit, I still have a fear nestling inside and it is dying, never having the opportunity to marry. I know you are saying; how can you have faith that God is going to bless you and then turn around and say you are in fear of something? I am human and as I grow stronger, my days allow me not think about it as much because the hustle and bustle of the day's journey has no time for fearful thinking. Yet at night, there comes a visit from doubt trying to confuse the opportunity's manifestation and has me questioning the arrival of my own possibilities. I laughed after typing, this thinking to myself as I admit I formed the perfect marriage with the atmosphere of words and I do not want the devil to play ring around the roses with my promises. I just want to be honest about the thoughts that have haunted me over the years. I always think on the day when I got the news from my mother that the doctors had given up on me. I then reminisce the words my mother still says to me when things get a little rocky, *"God did not leave you here for nothing,"* I know He has a plan, but why does it have to take so long? Well here is the answer. We may be asking for the wrong thing. As we reflect on our asking, know that if it is in His will, you know the rest. Have you ever thought about a feeling you got (discernment) that did not sit right with you and you changed your mind? God was protecting you from whatever it was and He did not want you to get involved.

We challenge our opportunities to see what it would be like, excited about the chance to do something spectacular; God did not ordain not knowing the ramifications. Research your motives, and ask yourself questions why do I want that job? Why does that man or woman want to marry you? Why do you want a new car? There is a reason for everything and I know as I was reading a passage ***in James 4:3; "When you ask, you do not receive, because you ask with wrong motives, that you may spend what you get on your pleasures."*** You have more to be concerned about if you are not paying, your tithes and offerings expecting increase in your pocketbook. You want a marriage but you are not ready to be a wife or a husband. I notice people are so excited about being married more than the ministry and work it takes to keep their union together. The Lord's Prayer states and we ask that His will be done on earth as it is in heaven, there is no doubt in believing that He can bring all that we hope and ask.

Are you serious with your prayers and believe that what you asked God for, He will do? In James 12:6-7 the word says, ***"Aren't five sparrows sold for two pennies? But God does not forget even one of them. In fact, he even counts every hair on your head! So don't be afraid. You are worth more than many sparrows."*** So why are we in fear of what may or may not happen? I decided to count it all joy when people reject me, hate on me, spitefully misuse me or even smile in my face after doing all the above. A trusting spirit is a winning spirit even when things do not go according to our plan. Remember everything works out for our good, not a need to satisfy fleshly desires but to trust God. Sin stops us from receiving what is rightfully ours in the first place. We desire the finer things and the love from that special someone along with every other opportunity that is again, rightfully ours. When was the last time you reconciled with your brother and apologized for what you did wrong towards him or forgave him for what was done unto you? Forgiveness is the biggest thing that will keep us in a state wondering if He heard us. ***John 15:7 "but if we are unforgiving, He will refuse our petitions before His altar (Matt. 18:35). Matthew 5:24 is says that when we fail to forgive others, this is cause for a failed request for His help, "leave your gift there in front of the altar. First go and be reconciled to your brother; then come and offer your gift."*** It is up to them to receive it or not, it is up to us to get what we deserve.

    Lastly, we must be patient. It is ironic that I am posting my daily scripture from The Book of Habakkuk on Facebook when I wrote this, who was a minor prophet, and in chapter one verse two, ***"How long, LORD, must I call for help, but you do not listen?"*** I know we all can identify with this. Praying and asking, crying until our head hurts but have we no idea that our true motives are for our asking. If He meant for me to be alone, it was for a reason. As I look back over the years raising my girls as a single mother, we have to be very careful whom we let in our homes around our children because we truly do not know who people are until they act out. My experience with molestation and rape caused my guard to be up at all, times including with those that spent the night. If God said it then this settles it…***"Do not be afraid, Daniel. Since the first day that you set your mind to gain understanding and to humble yourself before your God, your words were heard, and I have come in response to them" 10:12"*** After studying this, I learned that the very day Daniel asked he received but he did not receive right away. See God's timing is sovereign and we must be patient waiting and trust God. Good things come to those who wait. He knows what we need and I am believer of Him protecting us from things and people that we do not need in the first place.

My Hair

As you can see on the cover, I cut all of my hair off! Yes, I went natural in 2011 and it is very liberating. I decided to do a quick weave for a while but noticed something was missing from my life when it came to my tresses.

One of my dearest friends and stylist, Toya Adams was doing my hair for almost fifteen years until someone came between our friendship by lying and being deceitful, so I stopped going to her. I will admit as I told everyone else I was hurt. I felt the things that the bone carrier came back and told me were true regardless of our long-standing relationship. We share the same Alma Marta, 1991 alumni, class of Garinger High School and furthermore, being high school friends since we placed our flat feet on the soil. I will not go into all said but it is important to know we did not say anything to each other for two years. God would not even allow me and her to cross one another's path until one day at a funeral of a mutual friend and she saw me, came over, hugged my neck, and said, *"I was going to hug you no matter what and we need to talk."* I loved on her back in agreement. I had gotten to a point in my life where I wanted something softer and more sophisticated and it worked for a while. My cousin Donna Belk at Donna's Hair Gallery picked up where I left off with Toya. Since I had to move forward, I did not want the same look, I was trying something new. My cousin Ebony, the weeping

Wanda, in *Put It On Paper* started the natural process before me and kept talking about her experience, posting pictures and even YouTube tutorial on her natural hair journey. I finally decided in June of 2011 to take the rug off my head and let someone clip the last little bit of relaxer off my ends and start my journey. I went to a salon and paid eighty bucks for something I honestly could have done myself, but I had to learn. I coiled my hair until the length exceeded the definition I was looking for and then my daughter Pearl who is very creative with braids created beautiful styles for me. I soon got tired of that, you know you have run out of options when you start wearing Indian Braids, at least for me I did everything I wanted to do except put heat to my hair. I had damaged it enough over the years and so it was puff time, I slapped a band around it and wore it like the queen I am until I read it was not healthy to do that very often because of thinning around the edges. After my 41st birthday in October 2012, I knew it was time to make another change. I went to see my dear friend Quarvette Tillman, known as Quarter. He is and will always be my friend. Let me tell you about my friend. I remember in high school he always wanted a ride over his girlfriend's house and I would take him. The secret is why, he revealed to me, and we laughed like crazy just months ago. This nut was going to school from jail. He could have had me locked up. He is a very charismatic dude with a love for people. He loves to talk and he hates to see me leave when I have something to do, his reply is

"Oh you not hanging out with me for a little while today?" He is my friend for life and appreciates the wisdom he possesses. Many people do not know how to take him serious because he is silly, an all-American comedian, if you ask me. We talked about him being this way and how the character trait he has can work for him or against him. It will save you from being heartbroken, because hypothetically you can get results by asking questions sooner than wasting time finding out the answer later on because people do not know when to take someone with this personality serious, unless he or she says they is. I sat in his chair one day and said, *"Cut it off!"* Several times until the sound of the clippers took my afro down a notch. I love the opportunity to finish even quicker in the morning, because I can brush my teeth and my hair at same time. Shout out to the natural sisters rocking their styles and embracing the skin that makes you beautiful.

Disciplined DeVondia vs. The Alter Ego

This is the feud between who I am today and my alter ego who still want to stay there. There is a major difference between the praise and worship leader and the, you had better get out of my face before I tell you how I truly feel woman. Truth is, we have different mindsets, but share the same brain. I respond when people call my name according to how it sounds. If you have a cry for help, my response is immediate and on guard based for what my next is on the situation at hand. I know what to respond to and I definitely know how, however, there is a part of me that chooses to make more noise when she hears her name, Vonda. DeVondia, saved just like Vonda however, Vonda has a very vivid imagination and she wants badly to creep outside the shell and be with the world. Can I keep it real with you? Well, glad you allowed me to, not that you had a choice. We have to start being real about what we want and what we want to do. How will we break free if we do not admit and come face to face with our vices? Not that it is right to justify sin, but we need to compare our choices to possible outcomes when it comes to fleshly desires. At times, when it comes to what I used to do I miss the spontaneity of adventurous outcomes from my, I do not care situations. Judge me all you want, you do not have a Heaven or hell to put me. I am the one that says what you are thinking and fear anyone would know you felt that way. At times, I will go to the club and know there is nothing I am missing. The men are still eager for a big butt and a smile or a flat one with a pretty face. The females are thirsty for whatever they can get or stand around as if they got it like that and have no idea he just whispered in my ear. A part of me wants to fire off explicit language on Facebook to get my point across, but I know my vocabulary is better than that and I definitely know better. A major portion of me is tired of waiting on Mr. Do Right and wants to settle for Mr. Right Now. Yep, a bad boy with stimulating conversation and an opportunity to see what they may be like. Not too long ago, my good friend, Kim Williams and I, who I have been down with since R. Kelly, put the nickel on the needle engaged in some grown folks conversation. Silence invaded my kitchen, and I hollered out and said, *"This is what we used to do back in the day, sit back and listen to music, eat good food and talk about what we were going through with the men in our lives whether they were there wholeheartedly or a desire to feel a need."*

She screamed, *"YES!"*

I burst out laughing and immediately said, *"We cannot be doing this oh, no friend."* Feeling inadequate, not good enough or even too good for our own good was trying to seep in and we immediately stopped that drama from even taking up space. DeVondia wants love unconditionally with the ability to express her loving qualities without judgment on anyone's part. DeVondia yearns for lifelong commitments not part time indecisive opportunities that may or may not serve me well.

DeVondia has a clear vision on what is next, not discouraged and okay with disappointments and learns from mistakes. DeVondia feels what is hers belongs to her and she will go at any cost to make her destiny a major setup for the downfalls that were stacked against her.

Now Vonda on the other hand is a cool well-rounded individual who has the street smarts, wrapped in book smarts and drowning in common sense, but there is a side that still needs more taming. She is intrigued by the wondering eye, yet skeptical on the approach. She invites mystery and sends them away with dreams, all in the figure of her imagination, because the obedience of DeVondia overrides the possible scandals that would corrupt the best of them. I am not putting Vonda down because her vivid thoughts make the best stories to put on paper; just not lived out causing self-sabotage or broken relationships. Yet, some have created their truths. The war is more powerful than I am and the next chapter will explain even more.

The Spirit vs. The Flesh

I can scream my way through this part and hope you get everything from the loud noise that is getting ready to come from this chapter. Walking in The Spirit is an amazing feeling and I discovered before my diagnosis the importance of this. When things started changing and my attitude readjusted without my consent I knew there was a power greater than I but glory to God this was amazing work only God could perform. I would be slow to speak when someone would take me to a place where I knew I should have blanked out of my mind. We all know there is a part of us that feel that it is necessary to tell someone off. You will not feel right unless you do. The battle of my soul is forever between the Spirit and the flesh. We know there are many opportunities for freewill experiences. However when we are led by The Spirit we must submit to The Power that has the force we have no control except not to follow. My battle is my flesh! I pray and ask God to keep my mind, body and soul lined up with His word. I know there are enticements but also battles that I created and will continue to create on my own. I learned to stop giving the enemy power over my decisions to have sex or to curse someone out. The devil did not make me do it, I wanted to, period. However, God permits the enemy for whatever reason to start some faith increasing or failure to activate the power within us all. He gives us temptations, to learn from or to remain stuck on stupid. When

I noticed my love for sin, I was in Bible Study one night and my pastor spoke on not hating sin enough to flee from committing the act but loving it too much to not want to change the behavior that has us bound in the first place. I am candid about my temptations and I do not have to express my desires, I shared much of that with you already but I also have a mouth that will tear your face off. I am passionate about what I speak on and write about and anybody who gets the chance to hear me will know I will spit some wordplay off on you just because you are not doing what you are supposed to be doing. I am learning to channel my emotions more and more when it comes to what I feel others should or should not be doing. Here is an example: if you are a father or a mother and you decide to have a child and you neglect this child partially or fully you are trifling to me. Some may agree but there is a way to say it so it does not offend anyone, but help the process for the deadbeat becoming a better parent to their children. See I told you. I am as real as they come, well…let me be more transparent, I have a great personality and I am very humorous. Some of my jokes are not user-friendly by all and I love to laugh and at times, curse. There is no sweet sound in cursing so I try very hard not to make too much noise. I have this saying remember, *"I say what you're thinking and afraid for anyone else to know."* Forever embedded with language that will spin a man's head, make a woman mad to empowering them both at the same time. That is the flesh.

In the Spirit, I am more focused and quick to call on the name of Jesus. Just as fast as I smell the scent of a fine brother hanging a suit so perfectly and slow to speak when someone would have gotten a piece of Vonda but DeVondia allows the sweet presence of the Spirit to tame her weakness of her hungry flesh. In John 6:63, it is written, *"It is the spirit that quickeneth; the flesh profiteth nothing: the words that I speak unto you, they are spirit, and they are life."*

When I became a branch to the Vine, the true and living Vine that is more powerful than the fruit that hangs from it, I am responsible for the fruit I bear. It too will produce, good or evil, Becoming a new creature allowed my spirit to be new but my flesh, your flesh does not profit and Apostle Paul says our sin nature is in our flesh. In other words, we created to sin. As I ponder the rest of what I wanted to say I would leave you with this, I thank God I am who I am and I would not change my life for anything. I have been through some tough times, some out of my control and many were faults due to my own conscious decisions. Nevertheless, I am so glad I am not how I used to be. I am a piece of work and as long as I am hustling towards the mark, I am progressing in my transformation in being more of a woman that God has created me to be.

Fallen Angels

As you saw in the beginning, I honored two special young men by dedicating this book to them. The moment everyone dreads is a knock, call or a sound bite from the television about the killing of another black man. No one prepared for this news but in August 2012 was the first time I experienced this personally. My oldest daughter comes to my room and wakes me up to let me know NaNa is crying and she thinks something may be wrong with Popee. NaNa is what my kids call my mother and Popee is their grandfather. That Thursday night I went to bed early, I dozed off on The Braxton's Family Values. God knew I needed my rest. When I got the phone, my mom was crying it was not my dad, who had surgery a few days prior, it was Matto. *"Matto is dead, Matto is dead,"* she sobbed. All I could say was *"No!"* Numbness came across me. The sleep allowed my mind to work in ways it would not if I were tired. We could not leave my dad alone. He had got out the hospital and my granddaughter was born a few weeks prior by C-section. I brought my daughter over to Popee sit while I drove my mom up to High Point, NC to my favorite Aunt Geneva quicker than I ever had at one in the morning. I rode with angels camped around us trying hard not to let my issue with night vision get the best of me. Tears and bad eyesight is not a great combination, but the Lord saw fit for me to get up I-85 N in record time with no issues. As I traveled down

Main Street, I made a right on South College Street and to my left I saw crime scene tape and the flashing lights of the High Point Police. The Holy Spirit let me know he was there. I proceeded to my aunt's house and later we found out it was my Tootie laying there. My aunt is one of the coolest women in the world. When I realized she was so cool, she became my favorite. I can talk to her about any and everything and love spending time with her. When she let us know she was pregnant, I was the happiest girl in the world. I have a new little cousin to love on and babysit. I remember a time when I spent the summer with her I was babysitting Matto and fried a piece of croaker. Now croaker is the type of fish that my family loves to eat. My grandfather started the tradition going to the coast and catching fish bringing it back, and frying it up. When he would cook that croaker in that big black kettle at the church, pass me the mustard and some hot sauce, a grape soda and you can keep your napkin til I am done. Now my Aunt Genny is a fish frying Queen and she passed the torch on to me, her Fish Frying Princess. I love it. Well, someone knocked on the door and I left my piece of fish on the table to see who it was and when I got back, Matto had skint' my fish to the bone. He was very careful at almost 2 years old picking the bones. I started calling him "Tootie" and that was my nickname that stuck with him. December of 2011, I spoke at Duke University for World AIDS Day, stayed at my aunt's, and was able to see him. I loved hugging my little big cousin because I knew he loved me. He called one-day months later and told me he and Mimi, his girlfriend were coming to visit me. I was so excited to see them and enjoyed seeing him, not knowing that would be my last time seeing him walking and breathing. The most painful thing is how he died, a violent death with a gunshot wound to his head at point blank range. No mother should have to bury her child, we say, and it is a hard pill to swallow and we know that he is resting and do not have to worry about the cares of the world anymore. Just a little over a year later my aunt here in Charlotte, NC, Sonia lost her son to a violent death in July of 2013. My job had just run out at the health department and I got another job but the company said I was not a good fit for the company. God knew I needed to be there for my family and He knew I would. Working eight am to five pm would not go over well with a new job no matter the circumstance. Davion Najee Funderburk was a twenty-one year old graduate of Vance High School with a charming personality and was a big jokester. I experienced a reality that was a hurtful scene to see, him lying there with tubes in his mouth and a machine to breathe. The tears these women shed over the death of their sons are cries of remembrance. The shakiness in their voices when certain moments creep in allows their emotions to get the best of them without truly showing it. Black on Black crime is a serious issue in our community. We do not have to worry about the KKK killing us anymore because we are against one another. We need more black men stepping up to the plate and wrapping their arms around our fatherless children, especially their own. This was the most emotional piece of writing

I ever had to do, but I knew that I could not go any further without showing love to my cousins.

In loving memory of

Matto Ayim Nyiam 08/29/1982 – 08/16/2012

Davion Najee Funderburk 12/01/1991 – 07/12/2013

Why I Write

I write because it is stimulating, empowering and a therapeutic release from whatever tries to hold me in captivity. I love conversations and the reactions that it brings when the unexpected gives an expected expression from the pages my readers turn or scroll on my social sites. Every nine and a half minutes someone's diagnosed with HIV and the behaviors that allow the disease to enter in are some of the same others are playing with.

I love helping people save themselves from themselves. I had no one to tell me "*Vonda do not do that* or *Vonda you need to sit down somewhere and #GetchoLife*." No one put their foot down on my behavior but cheered me on because I was big bad Vonda. Are we really our sister's keeper? Real talk I do not blame any of my friends for what I chose to do with my mind, body and soul, however, I feel sound advice from a sister friend or even a stranger that knew I was a fool out here may have been a different outcome for me. Where would I be if I did not have HIV? This question posed after one of my speaking engagements. The young woman wanted to know would I still be doing something as powerful if it were not for the disease. I let her know everything I did before my disease prepared me for something great. So with or without I'm Trisha's daughter and I am bound to be greater than expected plus an added bonus I'm A King's Kid. I love to play with words because it allows me to secretly express myself to myself and uncover things I usually do not like to discuss. Dating since the diagnosis probably would be my biggest obstacle besides getting this weight off, but hey, it takes time. I get out what urks me; what disturbs me and what helps me by using personal experiences accompanied with witty humor and common sense, hoping that somebody gets it. I am not here to force change; I want to be the change I want people to see. Looking back, the naysayers had a lot to say and what was supposed to happen to me did not! While I have a chance, I promised God I would do my part in sharing my story in ways that were attractive, appropriate, fitting and making sure that He gets the glory because had it not been for Him, I would not be here. Writing allows me to go in a place that many have no idea how real the situation is. Either everything I write about has happened to me or I desired the opportunity. I used to try to live out my experiences but then I realized I was my experience. I was writing situations before they happened, inviting the universe in my thoughts and saturating the atmosphere with what I wanted to happen and fleeing because it was not what I imagined. Say for instance I may have been attracted to a person and I know I have no business going after a man but a part of me wanted to see if I still had it. See, after the diagnosis I became a problem within myself because I doubted my abilities to love, be loved, to please, be happy and I felt hopeless at times. Not knowing that when the time came, I would rejuvenate and my worth would find me complete when I wrapped my mind and heart around the thought of being worthy. My candid conversations tantalize the ears of my friends who are amused by my, tell it like it is, how it is going to be, and how, when, and where it is going to happen demeanor. I write on everything, the corner of newspapers, bill envelopes, my iPad, my note sections in my phone and my laptop. Wherever there is a space on a piece of paper I am writing on it and napkins are not exempt from ink either. I became aware of the things I would say and discuss with people, but with my close friends, I am VERY transparent. I thank God; Facebook came along after I changed because before I would have the wrong followers and friends for the erroneous reasons. Writing gives me a freedom that creates a safe expression in assisting women in my "Ladies!!!" post on Facebook. What many do not know, I honestly write this stuff from the heart because I have experienced what everyone has gone through, at least some of it anyway.

 I wake up early in the mornings, honey; the roosters do not have anything on me. I lie in bed meditating, praying, and then look at my Facebook timeline. Catching up on the post from over in the night or a specific post that stands out allows me to give the readers what God says posts. Sometimes I wake up and go hard because I'm so full of wordplay and I know someone needs to read the very words that God gives me to empower His people. Now I learned over the years that I could live a balanced life. I love to laugh and I love to see people smile.

Walking around with a sour face is so unattractive and the comments I receive on the beautiful smile and teeth I have I would not have it any other way. Being able to merge humor in to people who need a laugh encourages me. We have a lot of people that are suffering in silence and hiding behind conditions we have no power over but we can do our part by writing something whether it is on Facebook, Twitter or a simple text that brings a smile, makes one chuckle or shed a tear of joy. A simple I love you can make a big difference. I write because I can and the gift is a treasure I believe over the years will enhance and will allow me to touch even more lives. I encourage those who are interested in writing to put it on paper. There is so much to write about and even more to think about as I take my thoughts to my computer letting it flow is my outlet in helping someone in their go through. Try giving them an added boost in their already claimed and it is going to be a Good Day.

At times people may not like what I write because I speak very frankly on topics that women and even men should not mind reading, but get uncomfortable because their toes stepped on by their own vices. I will voice my opinion on not paying child support to sleeping with the enemy and it is not the person beside them but the one wrapped in the covers wishing they had a man. I cannot please everyone and I try very hard not to. My posts are to spark a change. It is the ultimate decision of the reader to make a conscious decision to make a life altering move that will take them out of their current space to a new place that will evolve them in keeping them striving for the more. I write because it allows me to dream with my eyes open. I do not take notes or build storyboards. I just let it flow. I turn on music. This is good to my soul. I love all genres of music from classical to R & B. Music brings me joy and I thank God every day for good music. I love writing while music is playing in the background with a nice glass of wine. The memories, intros to particular songs trigger something within and take me back to a moment and a feeling that can strike my keys on my Toshiba. Every time I hear Planet Rock, which is very seldom, it takes me back to the days of my youth when the old housing project in my city named Earle Village would have the block parties. Music would be playing, kids would be dancing and swaying while the older folks did their grown folks thing and it was all good olé clean family fun. There was no running from gunfire or dodging a hit in a brawl because somebody stepped on someone's shoes and started ego-tripping. Music at all times inspires a new book and ends a chapter, just like this one.

False Hope

I have set myself up thinking too hard on something or someone that had no bearing on my outcome. I hate when something happens for no reason, even though there is a reason, but no happening. I know I can be vulnerable at times and may get overly excited when it comes to astounding people and things. Anything I feel can bring hope and direction to my life is a plus, but when someone comes along and brings a smile, it is unforgettable. I said in *Put It On Paper "Anyone can make me laugh, but it takes a hell of a person to make me smile."* Men in many places approach me and this Facebook after dark my barber was asking me about one day is the same in the daytime I told him. Men will say the craziest things to get your attention. I had a chat one day with a person who just desired stimulating conversation. He just wanted someone to talk to and I desired the same. I was back into this communicating with men more openly without restrictions by their thoughts of me or my own thoughts of would I ever be in a wonderful relationship with the person meant for me. I no longer wanted to limit where I found love, but I knew the inbox was not the very place to keep it going either. The conversation came from the inbox to later in text messages. He knew exactly how to keep my mind stimulated and how to pose questions that would ponder a response with a needed smile and sometimes a loud "*Yes!*" I hollered saying, "*This is what I am talking about.*" He was a cool person to talk to and I decided to go see him, we had met years ago, but not on that level, this time was a mutual interest. I visited his place of business and had pleasant conversations on many things. After he finished putting his things the way he wanted them he came towards me and planted a kiss so good my knees began to buckled. When I tell you, I was mesmerized because I had not kissed in nearly a year and a half; my natural reaction was abruptly dismissing my presence. Caught off guard and was in no way ready for this type of affection from him. I thought I was. Was I wrong to feel good when he kissed me? Was I wrong to enjoy it as I returned the favor? All I could think about was how my body was feeling and how could I get to my car fast enough for no one to notice. I began to think logically about the situation he was no way ready for me nor was I ready for him. We just desired one another because we brought the energy we both anticipated, however, he had other plans that did not include me. Feeling wanted was a yearning of mine and he made me feel special, but I knew a part of me was not clean thoroughly because I wanted him and I knew he sought after me. This can tie into The Spirit vs The Flesh chapter because there is always a fight within trying to win against the other. Sadly, I did fall victim to temptation but it did allow me this, I am worthy of a kiss and I am deserving of great conversation without anything going further than the embracing of lips even though it caught me off guard. The opportunity brought hope that my king is somewhere out there, but I must not have false hope thinking that every man that plants a kiss wants to make it last forever or every hug wants me. No, I am not going to allow everybody in my space like that, but the mutual attraction allowed the chemistry to mix and yes, I enjoyed it. Something you need to understand is that everyone is seeking a desire when it comes to love and companionship and the importance of it all is recognizing what is real and what is fiction or fantasy. We all know that men and women can play the game well when it comes to getting what they want. Some lie and say they have a certain amount of income hoping to attract someone that likes to spend money and woo them on dollar signs; but what happens when the money runs out or the other person realizes there was no money in the first place. A Motive defined as *"An emotion, desire, physiological need, or similar impulse that acts as an incitement to action."* Succeeding at meeting someone's expectations with just words is very hard to do. You may be able to string them along for a little while, but what they were expecting is what they will expect. I did get a bit emotional for the person wanting to see him and even kiss him one more time; we both knew the best thing to do was not engaging further, that forcing intimacy based on feelings was a negative in the end. I knew immediately it was important not to be with him and not set myself up for failure. We can be our own worst let down, wanting something or someone so bad we fail to inspect the goods to make sure the expiration date is not near.

One night stands or in my case one afternoon kisses are just enough reasons for a happening to take place. Do not be ashamed to involve a self-exploration on what you desire and to see if it is worth it. In the end, it will be you, yourself and you.

Will you be okay after it has all said and done? Do not set yourself up for your own comeback. Love will find you when you least expect it. I am talking to myself, but if you are listening, believe what I feel. Waiting patiently is the only way to receive graciously the man God has designed for you.

My Appearance

Let me be the first to say that I love shoes and clothes. I love to look nice and I spend a pretty penny doing so. When you are a plus sized woman, you pay for the extra material. I have never been into high-end designer things because that is what they are to me, things. I never was the one to keep up with the Joneses, because really the Joneses are broke. Not all of them, but you will not see too many of them listed in Forbes or any other magazine acknowledging their wealth. Shopping was my therapy. When my daughter would act out in school after I had spent a lot on her I would go and shop to release the stress and look at receipts, in regards to what left over until next payday. I was an addict. I always had to have a pair of shoes and a new dress for church. Then one day a couple of years ago, God revealed something to me. "If I were to bless you my child I cannot trust you." This was a revelation for me because at one point I would get an outfit and a pair of shoes before I paid my tithes and offerings. I did not understand how important blessed was. Therefore, I put myself on restriction and made do with what I had and only purchased things maybe three times out of the year. I was amazed at what I had, and how I made it look good by changing the accessories and adding a different item instead of what I wore the time before. I dressed up to hide things. I had a saying "You will never know if I were going through anything unless I told you." I knew how to dress the part, but behind closed doors, I cried like a baby due to many reasons: unhealthy relationships, not being who I wanted to be and even not being able to be the person I truly felt I was. I wanted to say and do certain things that would not line up with the word of God, but I wanted to look Christ like and dress in a professional manner when I knew I was a hot mess. Now I can tell you this much, I knew when to sit down. As a former praise and worship member at my church it has been many times, I sat myself down because I refused to live any kind of way and stand before God at His alter trying to usher in the presence of God with tainted flesh. Yes, I know He can use the worst of us, but when it came to this sacred position, I wanted to be more than just singing I wanted to make a difference in the lives I ministered. Shoes, as I recant from Put It On Paper, is a statement I made in regards to "If your child went in your closet and put on your shoes would she be proud of the footsteps you set before her?" I started another change within because my walk had nothing to do with the shoes I wore. Vera Wang cannot get me in Heaven and calling on the name of Michael Kors will not save me from despair. I put more into what I looked like rather than what I was putting out. I wanted to be beneficial to the uplifting of the Kingdom of God not to the people who were not a part of it. I wanted to walk more as a woman of integrity and dress with the full armor without having to put on a façade that everything was everything.

I learned how to invest into my vision and make sure my marketing for my ministry was up to date and my home was inviting to my friends and family. I love the old saying, "It is not where you live but how you live" and I know I want to live according to a pure heart's desire not the world's expectation. Therefore, people, if you are dressing to impress, you are losing so many opportunities on the investment inside of you. You will never succeed trying to dress a part never meant to play. It is nothing wrong with treating yourself, but make sure you do it in decency and order.

Deadly Lesson

I have obtained a lot of knowledge over the years and one thing for sure I made some deadly decisions. One of them was not finishing school when I should have. I know everything in life is a process however, we can cause our own setbacks by the choices we make and I did that many times throughout my life. I recall going to school for various majors but never following through. Being in the classroom and not there mentally is not a prepared student. I stalked my affairs more than I concentrated in my books. I should have been further in my career than I was and I was killing the vision that was inside of me by not doing my part to succeed successfully. I had to release the state of "I can do it myself" mentality and start networking more with other likeminded people and striving towards dreams. Many hurt me promising to pay for my services until a caring individual told me years ago, create you a contract, stick with it and no negotiating. Thank you Delilah McDonald I will never forget that day you spoke life into me. People will pay for who and what they want.

  After that talk, I never missed what I never had. People thriving off the ideas that I spoke aloud, yet I neglected to pursue. In the midst of all of this, God allowed me to see people do what He had destined me to do. Every day I shed the dead skin of wanting a man in my Life, pretending that I want a godly man with a sinful nature rising inside of me. I avoided relationships because they easily bored me. Instead, I would seek refuge in food or men while pondering in my head, when would it be my turn again. One thing I can say about being in my flesh, I never took it upon myself to not inform my status to anyone or protect my partner and myself. It takes a lot to keep me stimulated and if I am not what I like to call edu-tained, I am ghost. Deadly decisions have cost me friendships, relationships, opportunities and even peace within, at times. People asked what life is like now so I decided to keep it just as real as I did before in my previous release; Life is blessed. I am on the other side of hurt, which is joy. I am on the other side of procrastination, which is about my Father's business. I am on the other side of forgiveness for all the things I self-inflicted that almost cost me my life. The only deadly lesson I care to learn from here on out is the reason for the letting go of the flesh that dies daily.

It is crucial to not murder of your own soul or the assailant of your vision. It is sad when someone else kills, steals and destroys but when we have a hand in our own demises its hell to pay to come back up. Stand strong in all things you do and trust God.

My Experience With AIDS

My experience is more like my deadly lesson. I wish many days that I never put myself in the position of contracting the disease that almost took my life. I thank God that He saved me because Lord only knows the reasons He decided to leave me here. I still question that at times. I have seen many die before me and I later found out that a friend from the hood had passed away. I also found out that someone questioned why I was not dead yet. Yes, can you believe the things that people say? People do not realize the hole they dig for me is big enough for them as well. That got under my skin for a couple of days like the guy saying he could not mess with me because of my diagnosis.

In October 2011, I began to wonder why I was not dead yet. I started crying because the Holy Spirit assured me that I had a purpose and there would be an expected end. I immediately had to shake that off, but it was killing me on the inside that anyone could be that insensitive. Well, my feelings did not regulate my response because I stated the truth and we know the truth shall set you free. God was not ready for me, plus He asked me to do something and He trusted me with the assignment. He knew I would stop smoking weed and cigarettes. He knew that I would stand before the masses and proclaim that He is a mighty God that saved a wrench like me from the hands of my own self-destruction. He knew I would humble myself eventually and not submit to worldly thinking when someone would bring me such information. He even knew I would mess up again. When I think back over the experience, it has truly established a different outlook on life itself.

By appreciating the aroma of things I love to smell, seeing the sight of beauty He created for us all to enjoy, and hearing the sounds of the birds in the wee hours of the mornings, I can inhale the serenades as they play sweet tunes and relax my feet in the grass of the morning dew. Being a survivor of this disease is not all bad, I must admit. Now, it does have its 'I wish it never happened to me' moments, do not get me wrong, I wish I never received the diagnosis. However, the process of this experience has gotten me through times I felt I could not. Even with my feelings on the brink of thinking, I cannot do this any longer. This experience taught me a valuable lesson on forgiveness. Forgiveness of others, including myself allowed things to work out for my good. I would sometimes sit and gaze out of my front and back windows to engage in a, what if I woke up from this dream and into a body not sold out by a disease that could have passed me by. I think to myself if one more person tells me, it could have been me, I will scream. Be glad it did not happen to you. I do not want to hear that. This is coming from a person who wishes it never happened. I remember when I used to say I was the chosen one for this appointed assignment. He did not give me the diagnosis, my choices did now, nevertheless, my assignment is clearly mine and mine alone. I guess it is a good way for people to reflect on how good God is that He passed them by, right.

I still cannot get used to it. I think people need to involve themselves in practicing the art of tact and diplomacy. I am definitely a better woman, worshipper, and friend and I must admit I'm not all the way cool with it, nevertheless, the hand which was dealt is mine to play, so what I chose to do is win, win, win…What you say?

Women Of Destiny

I have been a part of the women's conference committee at New Covenant Bibleway Church under the leadership of First Lady Evangelist Dorothy Beatty. I will admit this committee you want to be on. We all work well together and are open to one another's ideas. We are all willing to try new things, even if they do not turn out right, we are okay with it as a unit. This core group of women keeps me grounded in more ways than they could imagine. I thank this ministry of women who are faithful, organized, anointed and positioned to work for God. I have been a part of the committee for three years now and I am grateful for the lessons learned over the years. In 2011, the theme was Standing on the Promises, 2012's was Order My Steps and 2013's theme was Women of Destiny Discovering God's Purpose and Destiny for your Life. Every year, it is a grand time for the women of worth to come together and fellowship with one another. Kicking off the three day weekend with a Friday Night Live with a high time of praise and worship and a word that will lead us to the Saturday morning workout, breakfast and workshops facilitated by powerful women of God from various ministries in the community and closing out on Sunday with a powerful message and lovely feast and fellowship. Last year was no exception. "Discovering God's Destiny and Purpose for Your Life" was the subject theme for the conference and when I say I was realigned with my purpose from this conference I am grateful for the Spirit of God that was positioned properly within the speakers jumping off a friendly reminder of the promises God has given me. I will win. Unfortunately, I was not able to attend the Friday Night Kickoff due to school registration, but First Lady Beatty made sure I received a video of the blessed event the women experienced I headed out Saturday morning with my orange juice in tow to help assist with the breakfast. The kitchen was already humming with steam from a stainless steel pot awaiting the Quaker Oats Grits to tempt the hot water to a specific boil, bacon of all flavors, sausage, eggs, and croissants were just a few of the items being prepared as the Zumba instructor set the atmosphere for the morning fitness routine. First Lady is wonderful at putting together the structure of the workshops and the themes for each presenter. I love it that she gives us the opportunity to have input on what we want within each conference. My main objective was to get my zeal back. I was still sad about the killing of my cousin and then embarking on the one-year mark of my other cousin's death, my heart and mind filled with concerns of love for my aunts. I cannot imagine what they are going through, but I knew I needed to be about my Father's business because I have something to do as well. My assignment of motivating and inspiring women and girls is clear and it is my main objective.

The morning workshop began with a powerful woman of God who spoke on Abundant Living and the Importance of Living a Life of Abundance to why we are not. I felt a lot of it we knew however, the delivery helped me to relocate my reasons for not doing what I am destined to be because of my lack of living according to the plan He has for me. The next topic was "What Stands in my way in having a Closer Relationship with God." Honestly, I know it is my flesh; I was sitting in the conference rebuking a situation that has been trying me for weeks and praying I get the best out of the mess my life was getting ready to enter into if I had not been strong enough to reject the proposal. Being honest with me, myself and I was the reason for this book and sometimes I admit when things got out of hand or did not look good for me I neglected my prayers. I did not want to believe there was a future for me. Why would He bless a messed up woman with a message that seems no one wants to hear?

I challenged my position many times before this conference. I knew life meant to live, there would be curve balls out of my control, God was God all alone, and He needed no help from me. Yet I wanted to do it all and try to fix it, fix people, make people happy, say yes and do what asked of me without an attitude. I have no problem with chastisement but I knew that I needed to be sensitive to the Holy Spirit. This scripture was a blessing to me and it allowed me to see what I was doing was not in line with my mission; 1Timothy 5:13 *"Besides, they get into the habit of being idle and going about from house to house. And not only do they become idlers, but also busybodies who talk nonsense, saying things they ought not to."*

This was where I was in my mind; I was talking against my destiny, contemplating my reasons for moving forward or even killing it all together. I know I am nothing without God and I needed breath breathed back in me, I felt my life could not take another hit. I was tired of walking around strong for everyone else and no one to help with sorting out my own. I knew I could go to First Lady and any other woman of God, but here I was trying to fix it again. I forgave the individuals who did this hateful crime to my loved ones and caused the pain within my family's hearts, but theirs as well. A pain I do not want to experience. Life throws you different sizes of balls. When they come, prepared or not I decided I would rather swerve than being hit. Sometimes you just cannot dodge the opportunity.

My Hopes & Dreams

My hopes and dreams are the desires of my heart. I want to be distinctive in helping others to see the potential they possess at being successful in things they set their minds out to achieve. I want Complete Steps Coaching to be a staple in the community and internationally known to make a difference in the lives of women and girls. My hopes are to assist those who have a story to tell and guide them on a path to becoming a successful author. I want to instill in them to believe in their writings and be great at their beliefs.

My hope is to stand behind my brand and be the type of executive who is respected and able to hire others to have a position in either one of my companies so they too are empowered to move forward in whatever they decide as the motivation overflows unto them to be their own boss. My mission is still clear with The Rasberrirose Foundation Inc., to continue its plight in making sure that women and girls all over the country are aware of their behaviors that will put them at risk for contracting HIV. How to recognize self-love, obtain self-worth and walk in complete confidence towards knowing who they are and respecting who they will become.

My wish is to minister politely, yet radically the love for living and the passion for uplifting women and girls in making necessary changes in their lives at being better towards being greater than expected. My dreams are to fall in love with the one who will accept me for who I am and be excited about love and what it has to offer. I want the beautiful courtship, walks around the park, enjoying live entertainment and candlelight dinners, laughing at his jokes and smiling when he is not with me because he leaves an impression that he cares. I fantasize about a man who is intellectually inclined that makes me open my dictionary application on my electronic device to understand the love he speaks and feel the conditions of his emotions through his actions. I imagine a king that knows how to treat me without limitations or hesitation; owning the will to please the queen that he has selected just for him. Strangely enough, I believe he will be someone I know.

    I feel deeply that it will be someone I know already, very well to be honest, but when the time comes, I can smile to myself and say I knew it. I desire a more intimate relationship with God. To be secure in making decisions that will please Him and keep me grounded. I desire for a close knit within my family and more structured activities that will allow us all to get to know one another better and be free at having fun with life. My desire for the world is to be free of diseases, hatred and economic despair and loving one another with genuine hearts and smiles of acceptance. I desire to be free from what may try to trick me, tempt me and smart enough to not fall for the okie doke. You see we all have been vulnerable; I have shared intimately within myself and now with you. Continue…

Finishing What I Started

I had a strong desire for many years to go back to school but, I did not know what I wanted to focus on I did know it was still highly important for me to serve others and help them get to the next level of their lives. My job ended due to a grant not being refunded, so the department closed. I prayed as I discussed earlier. Being there for my family during their time of need gave me an advantage over those who worked. During the process of figuring out how I was going to make ends meet I discovered an online survey filling out application after application and after talking to a counselor she helped me confirm that it was indeed time to stop pussy footing around and get my degree. I researched some online colleges, but was not at all satisfied with the out of state tuition. It is a pleasure to have people that believe you are great, but also great at doing what I needed to do and that was going back to school and complete my assignment from whence I started 20 years ago. I decided to listen to the sound advice of a dear friend of mine, Natasha Fetterson, who felt I would be a great candidate for the adult degree program at Johnson C. Smith University. I stayed on their website intrigued by the next step, moved past looking for a job, and focused on going back to school instead. I knew I did not want to work for anyone else. I wanted to serve the people and by any means necessary, I was going to get my heart's desire. I met with an admissions counselor with the adult degree program, filled out the paper work, and went forth with the requirements. I sought out specific individuals who I thought would write me a letter of recommendation and was disappointed in their unwillingness to respect the timeframe or even remembering that they agreed to do so. I did not allow it to discourage me, I just moved passed the immediate distraction and contacted First Lady Dorothy Beatty and she and Pastor Beatty wrote my recommendation letter. I started with a fourteen credit hours and I am currently holding a 4.0 GPA.

I decided I wanted to pursue my Social Work degree, but have since changed my mind and I became highly interested in the Communication Arts degree instead. I started Johnson C. Smith University, August 2013 and I will admit I still was not doing my all focusing on my personal life as I should have, because I was consumed with succeeding my incomplete mark in my past, my degree. Blocking my blessings mentally with stinking thinking on what was not tangible in my life. I know how to shut it off and on when I want to, especially when my desires kick in. I had to refocus and connect with areas within my life that needed rejuvenation. As I prepared my pre-New Year's evaluation, I noticed my plans were evolving. I reintroduced my new self to my old self and living my life as if there was no tomorrow. Of course, I came up against some opposition. You know there are those that do not want to see you get ahead of them before they even try to make a move in the right direction, hating they did not do it first, sounds so familiar. It takes me to when my Pastor says, "You know when God tells you to testify and you don't." Then someone stands up and tells your testimony and you wish you would have.

It is important not allowing anyone to be a disturbance in anything He puts in you. I used to think it was a shame it took so long but as I know, is true; everything that I went through was simple agitation to get the assignment on course and moving according to His divine plan. I conquered the importance of advancing in my study habits and using my time wisely. Being a returning adult student took a lot of hard thinking and great support. I love the new friends I have grown to make a bond with at JCSU, especially my friend Toi Parks. She stays ready, my sidekick to the end. It is important to have someone in your life that is doing the same thing you are and Toi is that person. I chuckle at this because we had a Monday night football game televised on ESPN, The Carolina Panthers against the New England Patriots. I struggled with whether or not I was going to class. I even called and texted people to have them encourage me not to miss class. I decided my perfect attendance thus far and being in an accelerated program would be beneficial to me having my behind in my favorite seat in Psychology 101. I was a little perturbed because I wanted to be in the sea of Carolina Blue and Black. See, in 2004 I was on my so-called deathbed during the Super Bowl game my team, Carolina was against the Patriots. I could not enjoy the game; my mother had even put together an intimate Super Bowl party just for me. I lay there on the couch with my eyes closed but listening to the game. I was more tired and definitely weak as my defenseless body fighting to stay alive. I have tears now as I think about the goodness of God. His mercy is so great and I am glad about the journey. I have had my share of problems, but one thing for sure, any time my head was down I was in the right position to introduce prayer to that very situation He brought me out.

Stay focused on your dreams, allow your visions to manifest gracefully and never go off course due to the naysayers or a football game. You have nothing to prove, you simply have things to do. Get started, execute and succeed on purpose. It worked out for my good because we got out of class early and I was able to catch the game at the end of second quarter. Wink.

Ten Years Later

Tuesday morning at 9:15 am on the 9th day of December in 2003 was a day I will never forget. Here I am awake on a Tuesday morning ten years and one day later since I heard the words "Miss. Roseborough your test results came back great but I have one concern, your HIV test is positive." I was mentally prepared, but not physically trained how to process this announcement. I do not remember going to work the next day. I do not remember thanking God for waking me that day. I do not remember shouting through my pain because all I wanted to know was why, why me? I have a good heart, I remember saying. I know I cursed people out, but only when they pissed me off. I know I kept a clean house. I know I had a great paying job at the time, great benefits, I am a homeowner I remember thinking. I know I was fornicating with a man I had no business giving my mind, body and all to. What is going to happen to my kids? How will I explain this to them? My mind had questions and I did not know whom to ask. I had my best friends, but my restructured life disturbed by results entertained lack for conversations and I knew the ones I confided in did not feel me at all. How could they? My mama Lord how will I tell my mama. She raised me right from wrong. She had no idea her daughter was promiscuous. It was not a badge of honor sexually experienced because my love for love was desperate. Entertaining selfishly for the desires I craved fleshly, but on, December 10, 2013 I woke up with a Thank You God clothed in my right mind, activity of all my limbs and a heart that loves for all the right reasons. Yes, I still have a few choice words, but you have to push me to the limit in order for me to go completely there. I survived only by His grace and mercy. I was unsaved. Such a worldly creature, but I knew how to get to The Man who would right my wrongs. I continued smoking my weed and drinking my liquor, but I was numb from the belly button down. I stopped smoking the weed and drinking the liquor and the numbness went away. I did not want to have sex anymore; I lost that connection to embrace in the arms of the man I loved during that time because I wanted to make sure every man I had been with was not only ok, but also negative to the results. I wanted to have sex again, it was a feeling I got that let me know I needed to be needed and released from within. My kid's father knew they were straight but I had to tell them the news. Today, I have a peace with not knowing exactly who infected me. A big disturbance ravished my phone between someone I thought was my friend and even had the nerve to tell me "Bitch I hope you find out who gave you that shit." Oh it hurt like crazy, but you know what every dog has her day. I still do not know who he is and who I thought it was we had conversation and received proof that he was not the one. Am I worried? No, but I hope whoever he is, he is receiving care and being responsible with the woman he is with. I pray he is as happy as I am and enjoying life to the fullest.

Enjoying life, wow where should I start. I woke up one day realizing what I used to do I was not doing any longer and that was claiming my days and allowing my words to marry the atmosphere and blessed with bringing substance to each day. My days were going great and my nights were spectacular, but for them to be even better I needed to be accountable for my mind over the matters of my days.

Team Claim Your Days adopted to encourage my Family and friends on Twitter and Facebook About how their thoughts takes precedence over what they speak. I wanted more like the little girl in the AT&T commercial and I knew it would serve me right to allow my mind to get in tune with my outcomes before they made an appearance. Here it was 2013 and it was almost ten years later to the date that I received the news that changed my life. I wanted to do something very special for the ones who had journeyed along with me since day one. I wanted to bless media, community partners, and family and friends who have allowed my voice heard or simply wiped away my tears. Well things did not turn out the way I had envisioned but the ten year Celebration of Life Event was a spectacular Silver, Black and RED Affair that allowed me to party with a purpose. Also, raise money for my organization. Lord knows I could not do it alone and I appreciate the volunteers who helped me.

Each of them delved into a vision that was semi torn apart and helped to bring my vision to life. I decided after having a conversation with my cousin Ebony, who is my new best friend, that this will be an annual event to celebrate life and to do something for the organization at the same time. My hope is that it will be even better each year to show my appreciation to those who believe in my mission.

Mental Health Check

I can sit here and tell you what you want to hear, but if I am not real about anything I say or do, you will not respect the ministry been put forth in me. I was claiming my days and they were going oh so well. I said to The Lord one day aloud, Lord this feels so good to be in a great mood, appreciated, the sense of love I am getting, the advancement in my blessings and keeping me in a mindset of You got this when the weakest link would have given up. However, I know death is around the corner. Not physically, but I knew the enemy was coming in for the kill. The feeling that you get when it's too good to be true and you float anyway without a floatation device to keep your head from drowning and the tears from streaming because you feared this would happen, but mama never told you when. I was fluctuating in my weight. I had gained more than I lost and it was uncomfortable to sleep many nights. I was still in that mindset trying to convince many of you that I was holding it together, but was about to bust the seams out of my brain. I needed an outlet. I needed a way to diffuse the negativity that was beginning to come into my mind and allow me almost believe it. Not even sure if I trust what I believed or if anything I believed would actually happen. Doubt began to set in and my escape was the sweet taste of Moscato.

I limited my attention to anything except what mattered. During this time, it was about commemorating World AIDS Day and my Ten Year My Life Celebration Event. I wanted to live on purpose without restrictions and breathe without fault or criticism. Now was my time and it was nothing anyone could say or do to detour me from this place of peace. I decided to do something I was discouraged from doing. As I complete the process of writing, a book based on an unwanted experience because GOD said, *"DeVondia write your experiences in fiction form with a twist in order to help someone that may be going through what you have."* I am here to do His will. I am a non-traditional woman. I go against the grain of what others think, not that what people say is important, however, when it comes to what God says it does not matter at all. How dare I step into a field of no you better not write this book or say how it happened or change the scene of what should have been appeasing to man when I know God made this directive loud and clear. Every book I write is a source of healing and at the end of every chapter is a closer step towards deliverance. Fast forward to my doctor's appointment, I have not expressed this to anyone and I am being honest and true to you all at the same time. The virus showed its ugly head back up and I was not devastated at all. I knew what I was not doing and I knew what I needed to do. My doctor told me I was not being a very good patient and for me to be the voice of the community and the face of this disease I needed to do better so others could follow suit. I hate taking these medications twice a day with a passion, but in order for me to heal and be in an undetectable state, I will be obedient to the recommendations assigned by my care team. It did not meet my standards, but it is my lifestyle. I dare not turn my back on my children who need me. As long as God says so and not my own understanding or my lack of motivation to take the pills I must adhere. Through it all, I remained optimistic on achieving this obstacle so I can be the person, the woman God has set forth for me to be. Bright and early one morning, as I was lying in bed watching the news and scrolling through my Facebook time line I came upon this from my homeboy's post "Mindset is everything" I get this question all the time, "How do you handle it all?" I had to change my mindset. I could not wrap my mind around my scattered thoughts of the what, when, how and where's of my life. I knew this thing was bigger than I was and being an extrovert, I had to allow my aggressive demeanor to calm down and let God lead.

    I read Battlefield of the Mind and Power of a Praying Woman numerous times, but it did not matter until I changed my mindset and released a surrendering only God and I have a connection too. The "Why Me" affect needed to go, pondering on having a man, but "Doing Me" had to cease and the incorporation of prayer had to inform my hearts desires and match my actions. Mind over matter was my second to the greatest impact over my healing. Prayers of the righteous, God gets all the glory for it all because of Him, my life planned out to handle anything I brought my way and what He sees fit for me to go through. Without mind over matter, there would be no way of allowing the process to take its course. I am on this journey for a reason. I have said before and I will say again, God did not give me the disease. He gave me a purpose behind my pain and I am indeed smart enough to not allow anyone to make a profit off of me because I can provide for me and mine by being a light in darkness and a willing vessel.

This Is It

    I refuse to write another sequel to my life after AIDS. This is it. I decided this long before I wrote Put It On Paper. Frequently asked what life has been like since my diagnosis, just like yours. I pay bills, I struggle at times, I get my feelings hurt, things do not go according to plan and I eat, sleep, drink, and praise God. Rejected and got over it, I get upset, I may curse and I may not. I have to provide, so I hustle for mine the right way, I love the Carolina Panthers and LeBron James is my favorite NBA star. I adore great music and sink deep into the majestic sounds of instruments creating a melody so profound that I may even cry. I fill up my tank maybe every other week; I drive fast and slow down when I see the cops. I love my neighbors and the things I wish for are attainable. I am crazy enough to believe that love has already found me. I love my kids and my kids love me point-blank period.

Jermaine

My friend to the end likes Chucky and his Bride; even though, he is married to another woman and is happy, he is still a friend I can count on for great sound advice. Yes, I will continue to reference you to the pages of my first release, Put It On Paper so that you may keep in tune with where and how it all began. I am fascinated with the relationship we should have had in the first place and I know my place in his life now, friend. I value him and the extension of himself when I feel overwhelmed and sad at times. I may be the one that just calls when things are not going according to plan, bad friend, I am. It is great having a person intimate with for many years remain friends, even though things did not work out. Ladies we must know our role in the lives of men and not jump just because he appears to be the one. He just may be a fine friend with bootlegs and a contagious smile with a country boy demeanor that made you desire to experience him, but your role simply is friends. Stop jumping to conclusions and make each day one to know what his role is as well as yours. Emotions can lead you in the arms of someone that can hold you back from achieving your goals, diminishing your self-esteem and even shutting the outside world out because you mentally drained from moving faster than the heart can feel and mind thinks. I asked Jermaine at the end of 2013 how he felt I was doing with everything. It is because of him, Rasberrirose Foundation has a name and that I even put it on paper in the first place. Some women have men in their lives discouraging them when I had a friend who encouraged my talents and saw a vision parallel to my purpose.

    He told me I was doing a great job and he was proud of me but leave my personal thoughts off Facebook and put them in a book. *"No one will hire you to speak if you tell it all,"* He said. I thought about that and said to him, I will put it in a book because NoLimit Larry of Power 98 FM told me years ago, *"Don't give away what you can sell."* I was in the process of revamping my brand and gearing up for the New Year and this new release and Jermaine put something on my mind that I will always cherish. He told me I was a powerful woman and when DeVondia speaks, people listen. Now it was my turn to listen. I thank you Jermaine, for being a friend after all we went through, we remain friends.

The Day I Killed The Man Who Infected Me

In January of this year, my best friend Tiffany experienced the loss of her man to a violent death. It bothered me to think how she was going to handle it all. Knowing how strong she is, I worried about my friend dearly. I parked in a parking deck across from the church the day of the funeral. It seemed like a maze getting out of there: only to walk across the street. After almost walking around the entire building in heels, I was grateful to get my shoes under the nearest pew. Upon leaving the Spirit-filled home going service I walked across the street determined not to go the long way again, but make my way to my car smooth and quick. Once I reached the elevator I felt an inner body experience releasing outwards and the very words came out my mouth, 'This is the day I kill the man who infected me.' No, I did not commit murder or assault anyone nor did I attempt to, I was not talking about a man outside of myself; the man is me.

The woman that continued to hold on to a grudge that HIV/AIDS was going to be the death of my life, my purpose, my continued mission, and the possibility of love finding me. I got on that elevator alone with praise on my tongue thanking God for freeing me of a bondage that was whipping me in silence. You have to walk a mile in a pair of shoes especially designed for you in order to identify the feeling of chains that have fallen from me. I had long forgiven myself for making the careless mistake of being promiscuous and causing this tragedy, shame, and embarrassment on my family and friends, however the burden I carried silently was a fear of not being all that I am destined to be and that included falling in love and getting married. I knew I deserved just as much as anyone else did, but I could not bring myself to believing that this would reign true for me. I had a stronghold that was wrapping my mind like a rollercoaster at times, yet, I was as stable as the next. This freeing was a release of pressure that was gearing me up for a very special person that would enter my life, Me. It was finally time for me to open my arms wholeheartedly and embrace who, what and why I am. This great release allowed my innermost thoughts and feelings to vacate the premises without my permission and with all glory going to God.

    Finally, for a change I was free to think that all things were possible and I was not just reciting words trying to convince myself of it. Emotionally, I was not feeling that every person would be critical of my diagnosis and that spilling my life story immediately in fear of rejection was no longer a necessary conversation. It was time to do what my mother had told me a long time ago, *"Let people get to know you for who you are Vonda, not the disease."* I am a cool person if I do say so myself. Easier said than done when it comes to realizing not all the blame is on you, but for the most part, women usually left alone after the birth of a baby born out of wedlock. We are the ones who have to deal with the aftermath of being emotionally distraught after a terrible breakup. Honey I will say to you that I forbid in Jesus name you would never have to come on this side of the street just see by contracting HIV!

    I decided at the last minute not to give this last chapter a title. As I gaze through the window watching the wind blow, my plants wave beautifully back at me. Amazed by the wonders my life gave me and how I made it to this point, yet, I never underestimated how far I would go with the gifts and talents God has bestowed within me. Many have not been tapped into as of yet, but they are sure to come. I know I spoke a lot on many different things in my life over the past ten years since my diagnosis, but one thing for sure, I know I spoke a lot on being in a relationship more than anything Yes, we hear you are complete in Jesus, but He even wants for us to have a helpmate right? I posted on Facebook one day I wanted a man that looked like Jim Jones, from VH-1's Chrissy and Mr. Jones reality show, I wanted him to have the intellect of Tupac, a walk like Denzel and to love like Jesus.

    The Lord sent me the desires of my asking, a hot mess. It did not last; it was too terrible of a situation to write about. It was not worth the few weeks I thought would become something sweet. During the same time, I had a man trying me in my inbox. I knew him; he used to be my lawn person-years ago, but I never expected anything out of him except a well-kept yard at the time.

After we connected years later, he would say the sweetest things to me. Sending me nice things and leaving me with something many could not perfect and that was a smile. After numerous attempts of securing time with me, I avoided making too much of the interaction because I was stuck on Jim Jones and all of his counterparts. It was time for me to give myself a pep talk along with a silent prayer on how I was feeling emotionally. See, the individual I am speaking of did not meet my standards. Yes, I said it; listen to me people this was the biggest lesson besides parenthood I ever had to learn. It was the second week of January of this year when I realized that he was nice and he deserved a chance to get to know Vonda. As I was riding up I-85N with tears in my eyes crying out to God about the mess I had gotten myself in with the build a gent I had married the atmosphere. He said to me, *"I gave you the desires of your heart just to let you know that I hear you and that I can do all things. I gave you what you wanted and now I have what you need right before you and you are about to let it pass you by."* I began to tremble behind the wheel and asked Him immediately to please Lord humble my desires and relax my acceptance of this person, if he is the one, even if he is not allow me not to miss out when it is. *"How dare you have stipulations?"* He says in a voiceless reprimand. *"Knowing how you feel when people hold your situations against you why would you turn around and do the same?"* I instantaneously changed my mindset and pondered the very words over the next couple of days and then that following Saturday morning I was on my way to my nonprofit's volunteer breakfast and something nudged me to call him. I opened up my Facebook messenger and began to connect waiting on him to pick up. This deep orchestrated tone greeted me with a smile from afar and I muscled up the courage to ask him out to lunch after my volunteer breakfast meeting. The first thing he said to me was he did not have a car and my response was I do. My breakfast lasted longer than expected so I had run into my lunchtime with him and I was already full as a tick. I called him for his address and was on my way. When I pulled up, I saw a different man from the one who used to cut my grass. He looked smaller and his brown eyes were saying more without a word coming from his mouth. We headed for the Northlake Mall area and had our first date at Red Robin, known for their gourmet burgers and endless fries. I settled for a salad and sat nervously across from a man, finally. We engaged in some healthy conversation and he hit me with a line that melted my heart. "How long do I have you for today?" I smiled peacefully and asked how long did he need me for and he said, "Forever." I was done. We went to the movies and made a day of it. Not only is he a good man but he has manners that women of today are not getting because men are not giving it and women are not demanding it. He opens doors, pulls out chairs and assists with removing and putting my coat on. Chivalry is not dead. Me, being who I am, I explained to him about my stipulation because I loved a man with perfect teeth, can hang a suit, and all that other stuff that makes a man appealing. He understood and told me, *"I would get my teeth fixed because I want to be with you."* This melted my heart and made me again relax my desires and humble my acceptance even more. From that point on I would not care if he had no teeth in his mouth, he treats me better than every man I ever had put together and that is real talk. He is a hardworking man with a past and a blessed future. I saw potential across the table from a man with many talents and all he needed was a woman to cultivate his visions and foster his dreams. He told me the very words that will always be meaningful to me. *"All I want you to do is show me how it feels to be loved and excel in everything that God has for you."* This was a defining moment in my life and no amount of negativity could bring me down off cloud number nine. I had not been in a committed relationship in years. All of this was new to me. When he asked me to be his woman, he did not see HIV. He saw a beautiful woman who was smart, he wanted to get to know me better and we have been going strong ever since. His way of showing me he cares is like no other and it is important that we exemplify what real loves looks like, acts like and if there was a scratch and feel app we could allow them to get a touch of the amazing feelings we share. He is HIV negative and many may have thought how he could mess with me. Well, I Googled mess one day and got this definition, a dirty or untidy state of things or of a place. That is not me at all. Next, it said a situation or a state of affairs that is confused or full of difficulties, definitely not DeVondia Roseborough. When we announced, or should I say when he let the world know we were in a relationship, we had many to celebrate our newfound love affair and many liking, posting congratulations, patting us on the back and running up hugging have been discerned if it was genuine or not. I had a lot to let go of and one in particular was my insecurities of him truly wanting me for me and not for what I do or whom I knew. I needed clarity, so my prayers of course activated even more. He decided he wanted me to meet his mom, siblings, best friend and his cousins, and I must say my favorite thus far, is his grandmother, I knew it was for real. He gives me everything a woman deserves and I don't expect anything less, but the most powerful thing we give off is hope, hope for those who are struggling to allow love to find them, to keep it once it comes and to be okay with loving who their heart wants without the fear of what anyone thinks. For him, I am thankful and I am forever grateful for the opportunity to show the man of my dreams just what he asked but even more him returning the same. Do not give up on love because when the time comes and the right person comes along make sure you are ready to make every moment count.

What Is Next For DeVondia?

As I come to the final chapter in this book, I began to ponder what my next steps would be after my publication date. Immediately after this I will release my fourth book, *"Ladies!!! The #BeEncouraged Guide for Women of Color"* and later this year the second book under the Baptized N' Warm Milk Collection; Pastor B. Goode based on temptation of the flesh. I am excited about my role as a full-time student at Johnson C. Smith University and recently inducted into the Alpha Lambda Delta Honor Society. As I stated before, I will not release any more books on my life, but I will write fiction books based on experiences I have faced with a twist and also books for women with a focus on relationships and the importance of healthy self-esteem.

My mother may finally get her way because she has been telling me for years to write a children's book. Speaking, book signings, and consulting will be a continued journey, as I love respectfully and take a no-nonsense approach to getting everything I deserve and then some. I spoke with countless people over the years, expressing their concerns about their lives. I want to continue being the woman God has allowed me to be and a listening ear to those who value my expertise and my trustworthy ability to respect their innermost thoughts and feelings. The diagnosis changed my life forever and as you can see, it has not been all bad. I am just like you. I bleed the same color blood, I dance to music that makes me get up and groove, and I am free to give and receive and love without stipulations and the opinions of others. It has been a long ten years but I can say that it has all been worth it. I remember someone asking me if I had the chance to start over would I. Well, I would say no. If it had not been for my mistakes, I would not have grown to love the woman I am becoming. My love and I are embarking on a mission to bring encouragement and hope to those who feel love has no place in their lives. With our new unveiling of, "I'm Smart Boo". This slogan allows us to brand shirts, coffee mug, pens and bumper stickers to enforce the importance of healthy relationship choices. Soon we will branch off speaking to the masses. I see myself traveling a lot more since my youngest daughter is embarking upon her junior year at North Carolina Central University. It is time for mama to do her thing on full speed ahead with naps in between and a perfect nights rest. I see myself getting married, yes, it is a conversation, my love and I have often. I am just thankful that all the things that were stacked against me made me strong enough to knock down doors, create pathways and take the stairs when the elevator was out of order. I am a woman on the move with much more to do and my prayer has and will always be to finish all that He has for me before my head goes cold. To the person reading this book, please get tested for HIV and make sure you are in a healthy relationship with everyone you call family, friends, your man and your woman. Live your life to the fullest and make love to your dreams, never fantasize about your vision but manifest your potential with dignity and prayerfully execute every opportunity because it is yours. I thank God! I thank God! I thank God because if it had not been for Him on my side I know I would not be doing this. Until the next book smile on purpose and cast memories not misery, because no one wants an invite to your party anyway.

THE END

DeVondia Roseborough

www.ingramcontent.com/pod-product-compliance
Lightning Source LLC
Chambersburg PA
CBHW072021060426
42449CB00033B/1599